Nurse *to* Nurse

FULL-TEXT DOWNLOAD

ECG INTERPRETATION

FOLLOW THESE INSTRUCTIONS TO DOWNLOAD:

1) Use your Web browser to go to:
   http://www.mhnursetonurse.com

2) Register now

3) Fill in the required fields

4) Enter your unique registration code below

5) Download the software and sync into your handheld device

Code Listed Here

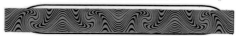

NOTE: BOOK IS NOT RETURNABLE ONCE SCRATCH-OFF IS REMOVED

Scratch off coating above to reveal your unique code to download your mobile device software.

See above for complete directions.

If you have any problems accessing your download, please email: techsolutions@mhedu.com

P/N 9780071592857
0071592857
part of set
ISBN 978-0-07-159283-3
MHID 0-07-159283-0

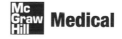

mcgraw-hillmedical.com

Nurse to Nurse
ECG
INTERPRETATION

Nurse to Nurse
ECG
INTERPRETATION

Peggy Jenkins, M.S., CAS, CCRN
Department of Nursing
Hartwick College
Oneonta, New York

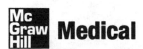

Medical

New York Chicago San Francisco Lisbon London Madrid Mexico City
Milan New Delhi San Juan Seoul Singapore Sydney Toronto

Nurse to Nurse: ECG Interpretation

Copyright © 2010 by The McGraw-Hill Companies, Inc. All rights reserved.
Printed in the United States of America. Except as permitted under the United
States copyright Act of 1976, no part of this publication may be reproduced or
distributed in any form or by any means, or stored in a data base or retrieval system, without the prior written permission of the publisher.

1 2 3 4 5 6 7 8 9 0   DOC/DOC   13 12 11 10 9

Set 978-0-07-159283-3; MHID 0-07-159283-0
Book 978-0-07-159284-0; MHID 0-07-159284-9
Card 978-0-07-159285-7; MHID 0-07-159285-7

This book was set in Berkeley Book by International Typesetting and Composition.
The editors were Joseph Morita and Karen Davis.
The production supervisor was Catherine H. Saggese.
Production management was provided by Deepti Narwat, International
Typesetting and Composition.
The book designer was Eve Siegel.
The cover designer was David Del' Accio.
The index was prepared by Kevin Broccoli.
RR Donnelley was printer and binder.

This book is printed on acid-free paper

Library of Congress Cataloging-in-Publication Data

Jenkins, Peggy (Peggy Jean)
    Nurse to nurse. ECG interpretation / Peggy Jenkins.
        p. ; cm.
    Includes bibliographical references and index.
    ISBN-13: 978-0-07-159283-3 (pbk. : alk. paper)
    ISBN-10: 0-07-159283-0 (pbk. : alk. paper)
    ISBN-13: 978-0-07-159283-3 (set)
    1. Electrocardiography.   2. Heart—Diseases—Nursing.   I. Title.
II. Title: ECG interpretation.
    [DNLM: 1. Electrocardiography—nursing.   2. Arrhythmias,
Cardiac—nursing.   WY 152.5 J52n 2009]
    RC683.5.E5J455 2009
    616.1'207547—dc22
                                                        2009017069

I dedicate this book to the loving support of my parents and three sons (Paul, Stephen, and Ryan)

who have inspired me to live my dreams.

Contents

Preface ix
Acknowledgments xiii

Chapter 1 Basic Principles of ECG
Interpretation 1

Chapter 2 Sinus Rhythms 27

Chapter 3 Atrial Rhythms 47

Chapter 4 Junctional Rhythms 83

Chapter 5 Ventricular Rhythms 117

Chapter 6 Atrioventricular Heart Blocks 163

Chapter 7 Helpful Hints to Ease
Interpretation 189

Chapter 8 Electrolyte ECG Changes 215

Chapter 9 Myocardial Infarction 251

Chapter 10 Pacemakers 281

Appendix A 303
B 305
C 307

Index 309

Preface

This pocket reference is appropriately sized to be able to be kept at the point-of-care to facilitate ease and accuracy in ECG interpretation at critical times in a patient's life. Attempting to find and use a reference on the unit at urgent and emergent times can be very difficult to achieve when the adrenalin is already flowing. Current practices of computers at the bedside are helping to keep nursing care at the bedside and decrease time and effort spent racing through the halls to find resources, collaborate with other departments, and document care. Instead of one shelf of textbooks on each unit situated next to the protocols, procedures, and infection control manual, a pocket reference is right where it's needed—in the nurse's pocket at the bedside ready for use. Resources readily available for use are absolutely necessary to promote time management in an era of a severe nursing shortage that is only anticipated to worsen over the next 20 years.

The purpose of this book is to make it easier to learn and remember the many different ECG rhythms found in clinical practice. Novice nurses, nurses transitioning from one field of practice to another, and hospital inservice programs may find this resource valuable for their practice. The methods used to promote learning include a purposeful approach to the use of the color red, organization of content in a consistent fashion for each rhythm (description, causes, assessments, interpretation criteria, and care measures), inclusion of ACLS guidelines and specific care measures, and an easier and new approach to how to interpret a real patient's ECG strip. Because many of us are visual learners, red is used to promote visual memory. Red print designates the differences between the interpretation criteria of a dysrhythmia and the characteristics of a normal rhythm. When learning (memorizing) the characteristics of a rhythm, remember the red! In addition, the color red is used to show the electrical conduction pathway in heart illustrations and the ECG rhythms on the strips. The heart illustrations depicting the electrical conduction pathway facilitate the understanding of why certain ECG features might be seen with each abnormal rhythm. Content is consistently presented in the same format, and in categories of three to five ideas to promote learning, as everyone has more difficulty in trying to remember long lists of content. A five-step approach is used to interpret the dysrhythmias. A practical comparison table at the end of the dysrhythmia chapters allows one to judge the similarities and differences of the rhythms within the chapter. Once the interpretation criteria for each rhythm has been learned, the question of "What do I do now?" has usually caused angst with many nurses. Chapter 7 presents a set of tables with guidelines for use to compare various characteristics of the rhythm depending on which criteria the nurse can most accurately identify. These tables and guidelines can make the task of deciding what rhythm the patient is experiencing a simple task! Rhythms may be compared based on any of these characteristics: origin site (sinus, atrial, junctional, ventricular, blocks), extrasystolic beats (PAC, PJC, PVC), rate (bradycardia versus tachycardia), rhythm (regular versus irregular), length of QRS I (wide versus narrow) or pulseless rhythms. Tables for each of the main content areas within chapters are presented for ease of use at the bedside when reading longer areas of text may not be possible due to time constraints. Because ECG interpretation is a skill that does not stand alone, causes, assessments, and care measures have been included for each rhythm, to make putting it all together at the bedside easier for the practicing nurse. ACLS guidelines for bradyarrhythmias, tachyarrhythmias, and pulseless rhythms are applied to appropriate rhythms and included in the Appendices for quick reference. Actions to take to care for patients with each rhythm are delineated under care measures including assessment, medications, education, and technological interventions.

Chapter 1 sets the scene with the basics behind electrocardiography and demonstrates the approach to attacking the interpretation of an ECG strip. Chapters 2 through 6 discuss the various dysrhythmias, with a chapter devoted to each of the main originating sites within the heart (sinus, atria, junctional tissue, ventricles, and heart blocks). Chapter 7 is unique! This chapter helps to put into practice what has been learned when studying the various rhythms. Tables are provided for easy comparison of the rhythms based on several different interpretation criteria. Because electrolyte imbalances are increasingly being recognized as contributing factors to the development of dysrhythmias, Chapter 8 is devoted to alterations in three main electrolytes that have an impact on the heart: potassium, magnesium, and calcium. Chapter 9 introduces three extra steps of 12-lead ECG interpretation to begin learning myocardial infarction interpretation. This chapter addresses the ECG changes associated with a myocardial ischemia, injury, and infarction and starts to differentiate between myocardial infarction sites (anterior, inferior, lateral, septal, and posterior). In-depth analysis of myocardial infarctions requires vector analysis and axis deviation, which is beyond the scope of this book. The last chapter addresses the ECG changes found in patients with pacemakers including characteristics of working pacemakers and malfunctioning pacemakers as well as types, modes of pacing, and care measures.

Special features in the book include "Tricks of the Trade," "Evidenced-Based Practice," "Clinical Alerts," and "Diversity Impact." Tricks of the Trade are small bubbles with ideas that make interpretation of the rhythms easier. Evidenced-Based Practice boxes describe recent research studies that apply to the content. Clinical Alerts are safety tidbits for either the patient or nurse. Diversity Impact is frequently used to address the cultural, developmental, gender-specific, or socioeconomic components related to a particular dysrhythmia. As a result of the format and organization of the book, I hope that you will find this textbook useful in your everyday practice until ECG interpretation becomes a natural and comfortable part of your care.

Acknowledgments

I would like to thank each of the following individuals/organizations for their contributions to making this textbook a reality. The expertise, talents, and patience of the illustrators are deeply appreciated for making the content come alive, visual, and more easily understandable. A picture is worth a thousand words! As a regional research and teaching health care agency, Bassett Healthcare supplied ECG strips to depict the rhythms described in the text. Without the ECG strips, the words would have very little meaning. Lou Priem spent hours upon hours reviewing the multiple renditions of text, discussing the content, and suggesting changes that were needed to promote clarity and accuracy. A huge thank you to all of you!

Illustrators

Eric Pierce, EMT-P
ECG Illustrator
Cardiovascular Technician:
Database Administrator
Bassett Healthcare
Cooperstown, New York

Stephen Jenkins
Heart Illustrator
Laurens Central School
Laurens, New York

Richard Benner, PhD
Professor of Chemistry
Hartwick College
Oneonta, New York

Contributor

ECG Strip Provider
Bassett Healthcare
Cooperstown, New York

Expert Reviewer

Edward Louis Priem, MD
Critical Care Physician
Bassett Healthcare
Cooperstown, New York

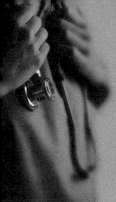

Chapter 1
BASIC PRINCIPLES OF ECG INTERPRETATION

Cardiac rhythm analysis may be accomplished informally via cardiac monitoring and more diagnostically via a 12-lead electrocardiogram (ECG). An electrocardiogram is a recording of waveforms that reflects the electrical activity of the heart. Cardiac monitoring can depict the electrical impulse flow between two leads at one time, while a 12-lead ECG can provide information about the electrical impulse flow from 12 different views of the heart.

DEPOLARIZATION AND REPOLARIZATION

As an electrical impulse flows through the heart, a process of depolarization and repolarization occurs with each beat of the heart. Depolarization is considered to be the action state, and repolarization is the resting state. During depolarization and repolarization, four main electrolytes (sodium, potassium, calcium, and chloride) move across the cardiac cell membrane. Five cycles of movement occur during this depolarization/repolarization process. In Phase 0 or rapid depolarization, an impulse is received by the cardiac cell that stimulates the rapid movement of sodium into the cell and a slower movement of calcium into the cell. In Phase 1 or early repolarization, the sodium channels close and sodium movement stops. In Phase 2 or the plateau phase, the calcium continues to move into the cell and potassium starts to move out of the cell. During Phase 3 or the rapid repolarization phase, the calcium channels close and potassium moves quickly out of the cell. Up until the middle of Phase 3, the cardiac cell is in an absolute refractory period and unable to respond to an electrical stimulus. At the end of Phase 3, a strong impulse could initiate a beat as the cell is now in its relative refractory period. While in Phase 4 or the resting phase, the sodium/potassium pump starts to return potassium intracellularly and move sodium extracellularly. At the end of this phase, the cell is ready to begin the process all over again. The process of depolarization and repolarization creates an electrical field and flow of electrical current that can be portrayed on an ECG.

CHARACTERISTICS OF CARDIAC CELLS

Cardiac cells have characteristics that make the heart function continuously and rhythmically. The five main characteristics are automaticity, excitability, conductivity, contractility, and refractoriness.

Automaticity

Automaticity is the ability of the cardiac muscle cells to initiate an electrical impulse without being stimulated by a nerve or other source. Most cells within the heart have this capability; yet the normal site of automaticity is the sinoatrial (SA) node. Normal electrolyte balance maintains the automaticity within the sinoatrial node. Lower levels of potassium and calcium may increase the automaticity of cardiac cells within other areas of the heart, leading to the development of extrasystolic beats or "funny-looking beats" that originate in sites other than the sinoatrial node.

Excitability

Excitability is the ability of the cardiac cells to respond to an electrical stimulus. At times, cardiac cells may become highly irritable or excitable from electrical, mechanical, or chemical sources. The increase in irritability leads to a lower stimulus threshold needed for the heart to contract. For example, the chemical effect of a low pO_2 or hypoxia may make the ventricular tissue more irritable or excitable.

Conductivity

Conductivity is the ability of cardiac cells to receive an electrical impulse and transmit the impulse to an adjacent cardiac cell. All cells within the heart have this capability due to the presence of intercalated discs located within the cardiac cell membrane. Conductivity of cardiac cells provides the mechanism for impulses to travel throughout the myocardium. So once the impulse is initiated through the automaticity feature of cardiac cells, now the impulse can travel throughout the myocardium. A couple of components that may affect the conductivity of the cardiac cells can be parasympathetic/sympathetic stimulation and medications. For example, parasympathetic stimulation can slow down the conductivity of the impulse, while sympathetic stimulation may speed up the conductivity of the impulse.

Contractility

Contractility is the ability of the myocardium to shorten its muscle fibers in response to the conducted electrical stimulus. The shortening of the muscle fibers results in contraction of the atria and the ventricles, producing forward movement of blood through the heart and into the body's periphery, generating a pulse. The strength of the contraction may be altered by positive or negative inotropic drugs, which increase or decrease the force of the muscle contraction. For example, digoxin is a positive inotropic agent that increases the force of contraction by inhibiting the sodium/potassium pump. Diltiazem is a negative inotropic agent that decreases the force of contraction by blocking the action of the calcium in the actin-myosin filaments of the muscle cells.

Refractoriness

The refractory period is the length of rest time needed after the depolarization period and contraction of the muscle. In cardiac cells, three refractory periods are differentiated to correspond with the heart's ability to respond to a subsequent electrical stimulus: absolute, relative, and supernormal. An absolute refractory period is the time period between the beginning of the QRS complex to the T wave peak, which envelops the initial phases of the cardiac action potential including Phases 0, 1, 2, and part of 3. During the absolute refractory period, the cardiac cell is totally unable to respond to an electrical stimulus with cellular depolarization or contraction. The relative refractory period occurs during the downward slope of the T wave, when some cardiac cells have repolarized, yet other cardiac cells are in the process of repolarization. At this point in time, cardiac cells can depolarize and immediately initiate another beat only when the electrical stimulus is much stronger than the usual electrical stimulation needed to create a beat. An example of a beat originating during this time period is a premature ventricular contraction with an R-on-T phenomenon. The supernormal refractory period occurs at the end of the T wave. During the supernormal period, a weaker electrical stimulus can initiate depolarization and cardiac contraction. Examples of the beats originating during the supernormal refractory period include extrasystolic beats such as premature atrial contractions, premature junctional contractions, and premature ventricular contractions.

MECHANICAL EVENTS

The waveforms seen on an ECG normally reflect simultaneous mechanical events. The presence of a P wave is associated with contraction of the atria. The presence of a QRS complex is associated with ventricular contraction while a T wave is associated with ventricular muscle relaxation. The electrical events associated with atrial relaxation are not visible on an ECG. The mechanical events and electrical events in combination determine the amount of blood leaving the left ventricle to be pumped into the aorta and throughout the vascular system of the body. The amount of blood ejected from the left ventricle per minute is called the cardiac output. A normal cardiac output is 4 to 8 L/min. The cardiac output equals the heart rate times the stroke volume. The stroke volume is the amount of blood ejected from the ventricles per minute—normally about 70 mL/beat. The stroke volume may be affected by three main factors: preload, afterload, and myocardial contractility. Preload is the ability of the myocardial muscle to stretch and contract at the end of diastole. Afterload is the amount of vascular resistance or pressure the heart needs to exert to push the blood out of the ventricular chambers into the pulmonary or systemic vascular system. Myocardial contractility is the force of ventricular contraction, which is dependent on the amount of stretch of the ventricular fibers.

CARDIOVASCULAR BLOOD FLOW

The heart is a muscular organ with three layers: endocardium (inner lining of the heart), myocardium (muscular layer), and epicardium (outer lining of the heart). Surrounding the heart is a thin membranous sac with approximately 5 to 30 mL of pericardial fluid called the pericardial sac. These tissues of the heart function to move the blood forward in a smooth contraction during the systolic phase of the cardiac action potential. The

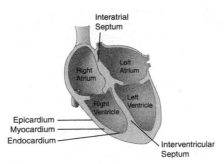

Figure 1-1   Heart anatomy.

forward movement of the blood forces the blood to move from the superior and inferior venae cavae to the right atrium through the tricuspid valve and into the right ventricle. Depolarization of the right ventricle moves the blood through the pulmonic valve into the pulmonary artery and out to the lungs. After oxygenation occurs in the pulmonary system, the blood returns to the heart via the pulmonary vein into the left atria. Depolarization of the left atria moves the blood through the mitral valve into the left ventricle. The left ventricle is considered to be the powerhouse of the heart, as it is responsible for moving the blood through the aortic valve out to the aorta and the remaining vessels within the body (Fig. 1-1).

CARDIAC REGULATION

The electrical conduction system of the heart is regulated by the autonomic nervous system. The autonomic nervous system is composed of the sympathetic and the parasympathetic nervous systems. The parasympathetic nervous system releases acetylcholine, which affects the heart by reducing the number of electrical impulses being initiated, thus decreasing the heart rate. Parasympathetic stimulation predominantly affects the SA and AV (atrioventricular) nodes. A reduced pulse rate may be caused by medications, such as beta blockers, and certain activities, such as vomiting, straining with bowel movements, and bladder distension. The sympathetic nervous system stimulation releases norepinephrine, which affects the heart by increasing the number of electrical impulses being initiated, thus elevating the heart rate. Sympathetic stimulation may affect all areas of the heart. An increased pulse rate may be caused by medications, such as nitrates and caffeine, and certain conditions, such as pain, hypoxia, and anxiety.

ELECTRICAL CONDUCTION PATHWAY OF THE HEART

As noted earlier, any cardiac cell has automaticity and the ability to initiate an impulse in the heart. Yet, the normal pacemaker site of the heart is the sinoatrial node. The conductivity of the heart normally follows an electrical pathway from the sinoatrial node through the interatrial pathway to the atrioventricular node to the bundle of His down the bundle branches to the Purkinje fibers (Fig. 1-2).

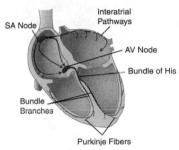

Figure 1-2   Normal conduction pathway of the heart.

Sinoatrial Node

The sinoatrial (SA) node is located in the upper posterior wall of the right atrium just distal to the opening from the superior vena cava. It is responsible for the normal pacemaker function of the heart. The SA node's automaticity initiates beats at a rate of 60 to 100 beats per minute (bpm) normally.

Interatrial and Internodal Pathways

The electrical impulse is normally conducted from the SA node through the interatrial pathway in the left atria to the AV node. The interatrial pathway in the left atria is also called the Bachmann bundle. The electrical impulse travels through the right atria via the anterior, middle, and posterior internodal pathways. These electrical pathways spread the impulse across the atrial muscle to the atrioventricular node.

Atrioventricular Node

The atrioventricular (AV) node is located in the right atrium behind the tricuspid valve. Junctional tissue surrounds the AV node. The AV node lacks automaticity and is unable to initiate an electrical impulse or heartbeat, but junctional tissue may initiate a rhythm with an inherent rate of 40 to 60 bpm. The AV node conducts the electrical impulse from the atria to the ventricles after delaying the transmission for approximately 0.04 seconds, which allows for the atria to contract and fill the ventricles.

Bundle of His

The electrical impulse travels rapidly from the AV node down the bundle of His, where the impulse splits into the right and left bundle branches.

Bundle Branches

The impulse moves down the right bundle branch along the interventricular septum and through the right ventricle. The impulse simultaneously moves down the left bundle branch along the interventricular septum and through the left ventricle. The bundle branch tissue may initiate an electrical impulse when the SA node and atrial tissue fail to pace the heart. The inherent rate of bundle branch impulses is 40 to 60 bpm.

Purkinje Fibers

The Purkinje fibers are located in the ventricular walls of the heart. The electrical impulse travels from the right and left bundle branches through the Purkinje fibers to the ventricular cells. The ventricular tissue may initiate an electrical impulse when the SA node, atrial tissue, and junctional tissue fail to pace the heart. The inherent rate of ventricular impulses is 20 to 40 bpm.

12-LEAD ECG: LIMB AND CHEST

A 12-lead ECG provides multiple electrical views of the heart along a frontal and a horizontal plane. All 12 leads are useful when diagnosing a myocardial infarction, but for most cardiac monitoring situations leads II, V_1, and V_6 will be typically viewed. Limb leads are obtained through the use of four electrodes and include the standard and the augmented leads. The four electrodes are placed on the right arm, right leg, left arm, and left leg. Six electrical views of the heart may be seen using these four electrodes: I, II, III, aVR, aVL, and aVF. The standard limb leads—lead I, lead II, and lead III— use the right arm, left arm, and left leg, respectively. The augmented limb leads include aVR, aVL, and aVF, and use all four electrodes. Augmented leads are so-named because of the need of the ECG machine to magnify the waveforms to obtain an adequate tracing. The limb leads view the electrical activity of the heart along a frontal plane, from the top of the heart to the bottom of the heart, or from the right to the left of the heart. Chest leads are obtained with the use of six additional leads placed along the wall of the left side of the chest; these are identified as V_1, V_2, V_3, V_4, V_5, and V_6. Chest leads or precordial leads view the heart along the horizontal plane or cross-section from front to back of the body.

ECG machines tend to print 3 seconds of each lead in a standardized format with three rows of four columns. Column one includes leads I, II, and III. Column two includes aVR, aVL, and aVF. Column three includes V_1, V_2, and V_3. Column four represents the remaining chest leads of V_4, V_5, and V_6. Typically, lead II flows along the base of the 12-lead ECG.

ECG PROCEDURE: CARDIAC MONITORING AND 12 LEADS

Cardiac monitoring allows for 24-hour visualization of the patient's electrical activity within the heart, but typically limits the views of the electrical activity to two views at any one time. A 12-lead ECG permits viewing of 12 electrical positions in the heart, but is a cumbersome method for 24-hour monitoring. When monitoring a patient's electrical impulse flow through the heart with either cardiac monitoring or a 12-lead ECG, proper placement of the electrodes becomes essential to obtain accurate data. When placing the electrode on the chest, make sure the gel of the electrode is located on the designated area and be less concerned with placement of the entire electrode.

Electrodes have better conduction when the patient's skin is washed and thoroughly dried before application of the electrode. Shaving hair from the planned electrode site will facilitate adhesion of the electrode to the skin.

Cardiac monitoring may be accomplished via a three- or five-lead system. A three-lead system includes a ground electrode plus a positive and negative electrode reflecting the limb leads on a 12-lead ECG. Any of the three limb leads may be read from this leadwire system, depending on how the operator adjusts the monitor settings (lead I, lead II, or lead III). Placement of the three-lead electrodes is displayed in Figure 1-3.

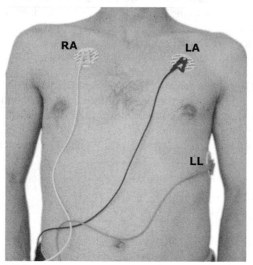

Figure 1-3   Three-leadwire electrode placement.

A second method of cardiac monitoring uses a five-leadwire system. The five-leadwire system allows for monitoring the limb leads and modified chest leads. Placement of the five-lead electrodes is shown in Figure 1-4. The five leadwires are color coded to improve accuracy of placement on the patient's chest: white (right arm), green (right leg), black (left arm), red (left leg), and

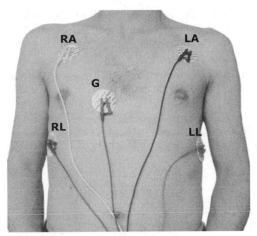

Figure 1-4   Five-leadwire electrode placement.

brown (fourth intercostal space near the right sternal border). Modified chest lead 1 (MCL$_1$) may be used by setting the monitor to use the brown ground lead as the positive electrode to simulate V$_1$. Using the left leg lead as the positive electrode and the left arm as the negative electrode with the right arm as the ground electrode, the monitor may read a modified chest lead 6 (MCL$_6$) similar to V$_6$. The modified chest leads can be beneficial in interpreting some dysrhythmias such as extrasystolic beats, identifying bundle branch blocks, and differentiating supraventricular tachycardia and ventricular tachycardia.

Tricks of the Trade

An easy way to remember placement of the color-coded electrodes for the five-leadwire system is "white on the upper right," "snow on trees" (white above green), "smoke above fire" (black above red), and "chocolate's close to the heart" (brown).

The 12-lead ECG provides the most thorough ability to interpret electrical activity within the heart. In a 12-lead ECG, an electrode is placed on each upper arm and lower leg to monitor the standard   leads (I, II, and III) and augmented leads (aVR, aVL, and aVF) along the frontal plane. In addition, chest leads may be used to evaluate the horizontal plane of electrical activity through assessment of V_1 to V_6. Placement of the electrodes on the arms, legs, and chest may be seen in Figure 1-5.

Location of the positive electrode for limb, augmented, and chest leads determines the view of the heart surface that may be

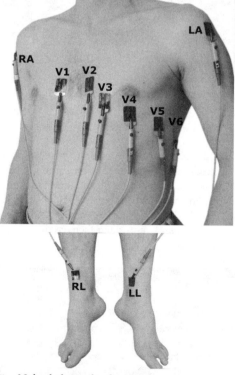

Figure 1-5   12-lead electrode placement.

observed in the ECG. For example, in lead I the positive electrode is located on the left arm which provides a view of the lateral surface of the left ventricle and displays a positively deflected R wave above the isoelectric line. The relationship of the limb, augmented, and chest lead placement site to the heart surface and ECG appearance is shown in Table 1-1.

Table 1-1   Relationship of Lead Placement Site to Heart Surface and ECG Appearance

	Lead	Positive Electrode Placement	View of Heart Surface	ECG Appearance
Standard Limb Leads	Lead I	Left arm	Lateral	QRS positive
	Lead II	Left leg	Inferior	P wave positive; QRS positive
	Lead III	Left leg	Inferior	P wave positive, negative or biphasic; QRS positive with lower amplitude in R wave than in lead II
Augmented Limb Leads	aVR	Right arm	None	P wave negative; QRS negative
	aVL	Left arm	Lateral	QRS neutral; neither predominantly positive or negative
	aVF	Left leg	Inferior	QRS upright

(*Continued*)

Table 1-1   Relationship of Lead Placement Site to Heart
Surface and ECG Appearance (*Continued*)

	Lead	Positive Electrode Placement	View of Heart Surface	ECG Appearance
Chest Leads	V_1	4th intercostal space on right side of sternum	Septum	P wave positive, negative, or biphasic; QRS negative
	V_2	4th intercostal space on left side of sternum	Septum	P wave positive, negative, or biphasic; QRS biphasic
	V_3	Midway between V_2 and V_4	Anterior	P waves upright; QRS biphasic
	V_4	5th intercostal space at the midclavicular line on the left	Anterior	P waves upright; QRS biphasic
	V_5	Midway between V_4 and V_6, level with V_4	Lateral	P waves upright; QRS upright
	V_6	Midaxillary line on left, level with V_4	Lateral	P waves upright; QRS upright

FIVE-STEP INTERPRETATION METHOD

The main rule to interpreting a cardiac rhythm on a monitoring strip or 12-lead ECG is to become boring and repetitive, and to consistently approach the interpretation using the same method. Become a "creature of habit!" A five-step approach is presented here and pulled through the discussions of each of the dysrhythmias to promote easy interpretation and to facilitate memory of the rhythms. When the dysrhythmias are discussed in subsequent chapters, the aspects of the rhythm which vary from normal sinus rhythm are highlighted in red to help with remembering the distinguishing features of the dysrhythmia. Lead II is used as the predominant interpretation lead for this textbook. Interpretation criteria and an ECG strip of normal sinus rhythm are shown here to demonstrate the five-step approach (see Figure 1-9).

1. Rhythm

Analysis of the regularity or irregularity of the rhythm needs to be assessed for the atria and the ventricles. Atrial regularity is evaluated by assessing the consistency of pattern between the P waves. See Figure 1-6 for waveform identification. Are the

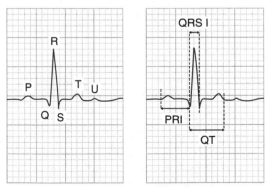

Figure 1-6   ECG waveforms and intervals.

P waves equidistant from each other? Ventricular regularity is evaluated by assessing the consistency of pattern between the R waves. Are the R waves equidistant from each other? Eyeballing the rhythm for regularity may be used initially, but will only help with "grossly" obvious changes in the rhythm. Two more helpful methods are the use of calipers or a paper technique. Calipers are a tool with two needle points hinged together. One needle point is placed at the peak of the P wave or R wave and the second needle point is placed at the peak of the subsequent P wave or R wave. Holding the needle points steady, the calipers are moved down the strip to evaluate the distance between peaks of other subsequent P waves or peaks of subsequent R waves. In regular rhythms the needle points will fall upon the peaks of the P waves for determining atrial regularity or the peaks of R waves for ventricular regularity. If the rhythm is atrially or ventricularly irregular, the needle points of the calipers will not fall at the peaks of the P waves or R waves. The paper technique is accomplished by taking a straight, clean edge of paper, lining it up with the peak of the P waves or R waves, marking on the edge of paper three P wave peaks in a row, moving the paper down to three subsequent P wave peaks, and determining if the P wave marks fit the next three P wave peaks. In regular rhythms, the P wave peak marks will match the subsequent P wave peaks. In irregular rhythms, the P wave markings will not match the location of the P wave peaks on the strip. Repeat the same process with the R waves to determine if the ventricles are beating regularly or irregularly.

2. Rate

Analysis of heart rate needs to be assessed for the atria and the ventricles. What is the atrial heart rate and what is the ventricular heart rate? The heart rates may be evaluated using three different methods: small box, large box, or "quick and dirty." The small box method is the most accurate, the large box method has the easiest math, and the "quick and dirty" method is used for irregular rhythms. On the ECG grid shown in Figure 1-7, the horizontal axis measures time.

A rapid estimation of rate can be performed using the count-down method. Once the number of small or large boxes has

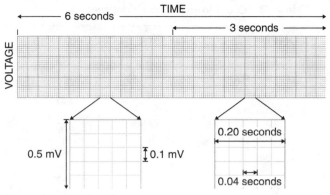

Figure 1-7   ECG grid measurements.

been counted between two sequential P waves or two sequential R waves, the rate can be estimated using the countdown method shown in Table 1-2 or memorizing 300, 150, 100, 75, 60, 50.

Table 1-2   Countdown Method

Large Boxes	Small Boxes	Heart Rate
1	5	300
	6	250
	7	214
	8	188
	9	167
2	10	150
	11	136
	12	125
	13	115
	14	107
3	15	100
	16	94
	17	88
	18	83
	19	79

(Continued)

Table 1-2   Countdown Method (*Continued*)

Large Boxes	Small Boxes	Heart Rate
4	20	75
	21	71
	22	68
	23	65
	24	63
5	25	60
	26	58
	27	56
	28	54
	29	52
6	30	50
	31	48
	32	47
	33	45
	34	44
7	35	43
	36	42
	37	41
	38	39
	39	38
8	40	37

Small Boxes

The small box method is performed by counting the number of small boxes between the peak of two sequential P waves for assessment of atrial rates, and the peak of two sequential R waves for assessment of ventricular rates. Divide the number of small boxes counted into 1,500 to obtain the number of atrial or ventricular beats per minute. For example, 15 small boxes between the peaks of two sequential R waves would give a heart rate of 100 bpm (1,500/15 = 100 bpm). See Figure 1-7.

Large Boxes

The large box method is performed by counting the number of large boxes between the peak of two sequential P waves for assessment of atrial rates, and the peak of two sequential R waves for assessment of ventricular rates. Divide the number of large boxes counted into 300 to obtain the number of atrial or ventricular beats per minute. For example, five large boxes between the peaks of two sequential R waves would give a heart rate of 60 bpm (300/5 = 60 bpm). See Figure 1-7.

"Quick and Dirty"

The quick and dirty method should be mainly used when the rhythm is irregular without "funny-looking beats" or extrasystolic beats present within the strip. A "funny-looking beat" or extrasystolic beat is a beat that originates outside the sinus node in the atrial, junctional, or ventricular tissue and occurs every once in a while within the patient's strip. The quick and dirty technique is done by counting the number of P waves within a 6-second section of the strip and multiplying that number by 10 to give the number of atrial beats per minute. The same technique may be applied to determining the ventricular rate by counting the number of R waves within a 6-second section of the strip and multiplying that number by 10 to give the number of ventricular beats per minute. This method gives an average heart rate. A 6-second strip is the time between three consecutive black lines at the top or bottom of the cardiac monitoring strip (Fig. 1-7). In an irregular rhythm such as in Figure 1-8, the ventricular heart rate is 70 bpm using the "quick and dirty" method.

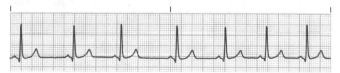

Figure 1-8   "Quick and dirty" assessment of irregular rhythm.

3. P Waves

Analysis of P waves needs to include recognition of a positive or negative deflection from the isoelectric line, consistency of shape, and the actual configuration of the P wave. First, does the

P wave have a positive deflection or extend above the isoelectric line? The isoelectric line is the baseline of the ECG typically located between the T wave and the P wave. A normal P wave is positively deflected or upright (see Fig. 1-6). Second, do all the P waves look alike? Normal P waves are consistent in shape throughout the strip. Third, what is the shape of the P wave? Normal P waves are round in shape. Other shapes of P waves can be notched, tented, inverted, or flattened. Fourth, what is the ratio of P waves to QRS complexes? The normal ratio of P waves to QRS complexes is one to one. Overall, normal P waves are considered to be upright, uniform, and round in a one-to-one ratio with QRS complexes.

4. PR Interval (PRI)

Analysis of the PR interval reflects the length of time taken for the impulse to travel through the AV node. The question to ask is how long is the PR interval? To measure the PR interval, count the number of small boxes between the beginning of the P wave and the beginning of the R wave. Again, one may use either calipers or a paper method. When using calipers, place one needle point of the calipers on the beginning of the P wave and one needle point of the calipers on the beginning of the R wave, hold the calipers steady and move the calipers to a lower point on the ECG strip to more clearly be able to count the number of boxes involved. The paper method involves placing a clean piece of paper under the rhythm, marking the beginning of the P wave and then marking the beginning of the R wave, and moving the paper to a lower point on the ECG strip to more clearly be able to count the number of boxes involved. One small box equals 0.04 seconds in time, and one large box equals 0.20 seconds in time. A normal PRI is 0.12 to 0.20 seconds (see Fig. 1-6).

5. QRS Interval (QRS I)

Analysis of the QRS interval reflects the length of time the impulse takes to depolarize the ventricles. In lead II, the Q wave is a downward deflection from the isoelectric line lasting less than 0.04 seconds and less than one-third the size of the R wave. The R wave is the first positive or upward waveform after the P wave, and the S wave is the subsequent downward waveform after the R wave. The question to ask is how long is the QRS interval? Again, using calipers or the paper technique, the QRS interval may be measured by marking the beginning of the Q wave to the beginning of the S wave, moving to a lower point on the ECG strip, and counting the number of boxes involved. A normal QRS interval is less than 0.12 seconds. The amplitude or voltage of the R wave is much higher than the P wave because the greater muscle mass in the ventricles can create a larger electrical potential. The amplitude of the R wave can be measured in millivolts on the vertical axis of the ECG grid. Each small box on the vertical axis equals 0.1 mV and every large box on the vertical axis equals 0.5 mV (see Fig. 1-6).

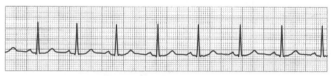

Figure 1-9   Normal sinus rhythm.

Normal Sinus Rhythm Interpretation Criteria

1. Rhythm: regular
2. Rate: 60–100 bpm
3. P wave: upright, uniform, and round in a 1:1 ratio
4. PRI: 0.12–0.20 sec
5. QRS I: less than 0.12 sec

The five-step approach will typically permit ease of interpretation of the many dysrhythmias discussed in this textbook. Keeping a routine to interpreting rhythms makes the skill to be learned similar to tying one's shoes—one step after another. Additional observations are useful for interpreting electrolyte, medication, and myocardial damage.

T Wave

A T wave reflects ventricular repolarization or ventricular muscle relaxation. The T wave is usually upright in leads with an upright R wave, round and slightly asymmetrical with a more gradual slope on the first half of the wave than the second half of the wave. The T wave typically flows in the same direction as the R wave (see Fig. 1-6). Changes in T wave configuration may be seen from electrolyte imbalances, medications, and pulmonary and cardiac issues. For example, an elevated potassium level may cause the T wave to become tented and large; while in myocardial ischemia the T wave may initially be tented, advance to a flattened state, and then become inverted in the leads associated with the myocardial damage.

U Wave

The electrical physiology behind a U wave is not clearly understood. A U wave is a small upright round wave in lead II seen after the T wave and before the next P wave. Although U waves have been seen in normal individuals, the presence of a U wave is more commonly associated with hypokalemia or the administration of medications such as amiodarone or digoxin (see Fig. 1-6).

QT Interval

An interval of time called the QT interval may be measured to reflect the length of time from the beginning of ventricular depolarization to the end of ventricular repolarization, or from the beginning of the Q wave to the end of the T wave. The QT interval is usually called a corrected QT interval or a QTc, because the QT interval is mathematically derived. A normal QT interval varies by multiple factors including gender, heart rate, and age. The measurement of the QT interval is performed by measuring the distance between two sequential R waves and dividing by two. The second step is to measure the QT interval (Fig. 1-6). A normal QTc is less than one-half of the R-to-R interval (R–R interval), with a borderline issue considered to be about equal to the R–R interval, and an abnormal QTc measuring greater than one-half of the R–R interval. A shortened QT interval may be seen in patients with hypercalcemia, and a prolonged QT interval may be observed in hypocalcemia or with administration of many drugs such as sotalol, phenothiazines, and quinolone antibiotics. A danger associated with prolonged QT intervals is a risk for a more dangerous ventricular rhythm, Torsades de pointes. A QTc of greater than 0.44 second is typically viewed as a concern.

BASIS OF DYSRHYTHMIAS

Dysrhythmias may occur in the SA node, atrial tissue, junctional tissue, AV node, or ventricular tissue. The dysrhythmia may evolve from one of several issues related to electrical impulse flow. The five main types of issues are disturbances with electrical conduction, escape beats/rhythms, enhanced automaticity, reentry mechanisms, and triggered activity. Conduction disturbances are dysrhythmias that occur due to delays or complete blocks of transmission of the electrical impulses such as with AV blocks. Escape rhythms are beats that originate when the rhythm slows down to a point that the atrial, junctional, or ventricular tissue initiates a beat or rhythm at the inherent rate of that tissue. For example, junctional tissue beats at an inherent rate of 40 to 60 bpm (junctional escape rhythm) and ventricular tissue beats at an inherent rate of 20 to 40 bpm (idioventricular rhythm). Enhanced automaticity is the development of a pacemaker site in the atrial, junctional, or ventricular tissue from spontaneous depolarization in those cells or from firing in one of those tissues that overrides the rate of the SA node. Rhythms that may occur from enhanced automaticity are premature atrial contractions, premature junctional contractions, premature ventricular contractions, atrial flutter, atrial fibrillation, junctional tachycardia, ventricular tachycardia, and ventricular fibrillation. Reentry mechanisms occurs when an electrical impulse circuits back onto itself through a circular conduction route and evolves when the original electrical impulse is slowed or completely blocked from transmitting in its usual pathway. The slowing or complete block of electrical impulse flow results in the impulse circuiting back into the recently depolarized cardiac cells from the initial normal electrical impulse. Reentry mechanisms are rhythms that evolve when electrical impulses are generated during the repolarization of the cardiac cells such as atrial flutter, AV nodal reentrant tachycardia, and many ventricular tachycardias. Triggered activity is due to automaticity of cardiac cells during the repolarization stage in response to a stimulus which causes depolarization. Often referred to as afterdepolarizations, these beats originate from atrial, junctional, and ventricular tissue as single beats, couplets, salvos, and/or runs. Rhythms developing from triggered activity include extrasystolic beats or sustained rhythms such as atrial tachycardia or ventricular tachycardia.

ARTIFACT

When assessing an ECG or cardiac monitoring strip, recognition of patient and monitoring issues becomes essential in an accurate interpretation. Several forms of interference can make waveforms difficult to interpret, such as artifact from patient movement, 60-cycle interference, a wandering baseline, and flatline artifact. Patients connected to cardiac monitoring or a 12-lead ECG can alter the characteristics of the waveforms through movement as simple as washing their face or turning the page of a book (Fig. 1-10). The waveforms created from patient movement may be mistakenly interpreted as ventricular tachycardia, which is the reason to remember to always assess the patient. Sixty-cycle interference may be sensed by the electrodes when leakage from electrically powered equipment occurs. The cardiac telemetry strip may show a QRS wave, but an indistinguishable P wave and isoelectric line. Electrical interference may occur with excessively moist skin, dried conducting gel on the electrode pads, or placement of electrodes in hairy areas (Fig. 1-11). A wandering baseline may appear if the electrodes have been placed near the patient's diaphragm or if the electrode contact with the skin is not intact (Fig. 1-12). A flat line or no baseline may appear when the patient becomes disconnected to the leadwires or has a leadwire failure or dry electrode gel (Fig. 1-13).

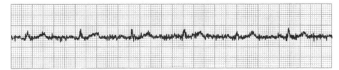

Figure 1-10   Muscular artifact.

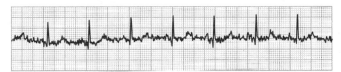

Figure 1-11   60-Cycle electrical interference.

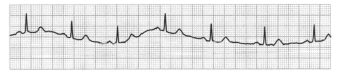

Figure 1-12   Wandering baseline.

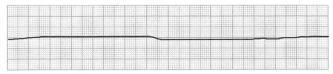

Figure 1-13   Flatline artifact.

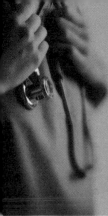

Chapter 2
SINUS RHYTHMS

A sinus rhythm is initiated in the sinoatrial (SA) node of the heart. In sinus rhythms, each beat follows the normal conduction system by traveling from the SA node through the atrial pathway to the atrioventricular (AV) junctional tissue, down the bundle of His, and out through the Purkinje fibers. A hallmark sign of a sinus rhythm is an upright, uniform, and roundly shaped P wave.

NORMAL SINUS RHYTHM

Normal sinus rhythm (NSR) is initiated by the SA node at a rate of 60 to100 beats per minute (bpm). Each beat of this rhythm follows the normal conduction system by traveling from the SA node through the atrial pathway to the AV junctional tissue, down the bundle of His, and out through the Purkinje fibers. This leads to atrial followed by ventricular depolarization of the myocardial cells (Figs. 2-1 and 2-2).

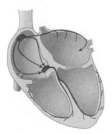

Figure 2-1   Normal conduction pathway in normal sinus rhythm.

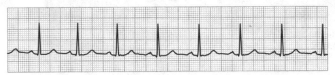

Figure 2-2   Normal sinus rhythm.

Normal Sinus Rhythm Interpretation Criteria

1. Rhythm: regular
2. Rate: 60–100 bpm
3. P wave: upright, uniform, and round in a 1:1 ratio
4. PRI: 0.12–0.20 sec
5. QRS I: less than 0.12 sec

SINUS BRADYCARDIA

Sinus bradycardia (SB) is a rhythm initiated by the SA node at a rate less than 60 bpm. Each beat of this rhythm follows the normal conduction system by traveling from the SA node through the atrial pathway to the AV junctional tissue, down the bundle of His, and out through the Purkinje fibers, leading to atrial followed by ventricular depolarization of the myocardial cells (Figs. 2-3 and 2-4).

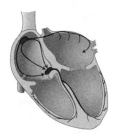

Figure 2-3   Normal conduction pathway in sinus bradycardia.

Diversity Impact

Sinus bradycardia is rarely seen in children, but when present in ill children indicates a poor prognosis. In adults, sinus bradycardia is usually tolerated well until heart rate moves below 45 bpm.

Sinus Bradycardia Causes

The general principles behind the cause of sinus bradycardia are primarily related to a vagus nerve stimulation of the parasympathetic nervous system or blockage of the sympathetic nervous system response, SA node disease, and higher stroke volumes per beat in endurance athletes. More today than in the past, sinus bradycardia may be related to medication administration, particularly beta blockers.

Sinus Bradycardia Causes

- Vagal stimulation
  - Sleep
  - Straining with bowel movements/bowel or bladder distension
  - Vomiting
  - Coughing/sneezing
  - Carotid sinus massage
    - Purposeful treatment for supraventricular tachycardia
    - Behavioral—tight collars around neck/strong water spray in shower on carotid artery
- Drug-related response
  - Beta blockers
  - Calcium channel blockers
  - Cardiac glycosides (digoxin)
  - Amiodarone

- Disease-related response
  - Inferior and posterior wall myocardial infarctions
  - Anorexia nervosa
  - Hypothyroidism
  - Hypothermia
  - Hyperkalemia

Sinus Bradycardia Assessments

Sinus bradycardia is usually asymptomatic. BUT, remember cardiac output equals heart rate times stroke volume (CO = HR × SV). Therefore, a significant decrease in heart rate can decrease the cardiac output and decrease the blood supply to the coronary arteries. Chest discomfort or chest pain may result when the cardiac demand for oxygen is unable to be met related to the decreased cardiac output. A decreased level of consciousness may result from decreased cardiac output causing reduced blood flow to the brain. Hypotension and bradycardia in acute inferior myocardial infarcted patients may be transient, volume-related, or indicate a poor prognosis.

Sinus Bradycardia Assessments

- Usually asymptomatic unless heart rate less than 45 bpm
- Chest pain
- Syncope/hypotension
- Dyspnea
- Decreased level of consciousness

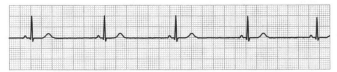

Figure 2-4 Sinus bradycardia.

Sinus Bradycardia Interpretation Criteria

1. Rhythm: regular, may be slightly irregular
2. Rate: less than 60 bpm
3. P wave: upright, uniform, and round in a 1:1 ratio
4. PRI: between 0.12–0.20 sec
   QRS I: less than 0.12 sec

Review Question

What criterion distinguishes sinus bradycardia from NSR?_____

[Heart rate less than 60 bpm]

Sinus Bradycardia Care Measures

When sinus bradycardia is found, the first step is to identify the effect of the rhythm on the patient's clinical signs and symptoms. If the rhythm is asymptomatic, determine and treat the cause, such as initiating a constipation protocol for constipation to prevent straining for a bowel movement, administering antiemetics for vomiting, discontinuing the causative drug (beta blockers, calcium channel blockers, amiodarone, or digoxin), and treating the underlying disease (e.g., administer levothyroxine for hypothyroidism). When the rhythm is symptomatic, further treatment is needed. Atropine is considered to be the drug of choice, at a dose of 0.5 mg IV up to a total dose of 3 mg. Atropine blocks the cardiac muscarinic receptors, which prevents parasympathetic nervous stimulation in the heart. If the first dose of atropine is unsuccessful, repeat doses may be administered every 3 minutes. A second measure is to initiate transcutaneous pacing, which delivers electrical impulses through the skin to cause depolarization and then contraction of the myocardium. If transcutaneous pacing is ineffective, try epinephrine at 2 to 10 µg/min or dopamine at 2 to 10 µg/kg/min while preparing for transvenous pacing (AHA, 2005). A recommendation is to follow the bradycardia algorithm suggested by the American Heart Association. See Appendix A.

Sinus Bradycardia Care Measures

- Assess impact of the rhythm on the patient's clinical signs and symptoms
- Treat the cause
- Asymptomatic: no treatment needed
- Symptomatic
  — Oxygen
  — IV access
  — Atropine
  — Transcutaneous pacing
  — Epinephrine or dopamine

(Reprinted with permission from Field JM: Advanced Cardiovascular Life Support: Provider Manual;2006:81. Dallus, Texas.)

SINUS TACHYCARDIA (ST)

Sinus tachycardia (ST) is a rhythm initiated by the SA node at a rate that ranges from 101 to 180 bpm. Each beat of this rhythm follows the normal conduction system by traveling from the SA node through the atrial pathway to the AV junctional tissue, down the bundle of His, and out through the Purkinje fibers, leading to atrial followed by ventricular depolarization of the myocardial cells (Figs. 2-5 and 2-6).

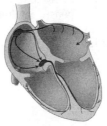

Figure 2-5   Normal conduction pathway in sinus tachycardia.

Diversity Impact

Determination of sinus tachycardia is dependent on what is considered normal for the individual's age, and is usually defined as a persistent and significant elevation in heart rate. For example, crying and discomfort in infants may transiently raise the heart rate greater than the normal rate for an infant, which is 100 to 160 bpm. Sinus tachycardia for an infant would be defined as a heart rate greater than 200 bpm.

Sinus Tachycardia Causes

The general causes of sinus tachycardia are sympathetic nervous system (SNS) stimulation and increased body temperature. Multiple events produce the release of catecholamines, leading to SNS stimulation, which causes the heart rate to race. Tachycardia may be from physiologic or pathophysiologic causes. At times, higher heart rates may be a compensatory mechanism and physiologically assist the patient to maintain cardiac output, such as with exercise. Actual stimulation of the SNS, from any form of increased exercise or the effects of drug therapy, may raise the heart rate. An increase in body temperature of 1 degree Celsius raises the heart rate approximately 18 bpm, while an increase of 1 degree Fahrenheit raises the heart rate approximately 10 bpm up to a temperature of 105°F. Pathophysiologic responses resulting in tachycardia may be seen in late heart failure and shock when the body decompensates and the elevated heart rate greatly reduces the ventricular filling time, leading to a decreased cardiac output.

Sinus Tachycardia Causes

- Normal response
  — Exercise
  — Pain
  — Fever
  — Sexual intercourse
  — Fear/anxiety/stress
- Substance-related response
  — Lifestyle-related response
    ▪ Caffeine
    ▪ Alcohol
    ▪ Nicotine
    ▪ Marijuana, ecstasy, cocaine
  — Drug-related response
    ▪ Epinephrine
    ▪ Atropine
    ▪ Dopamine/dobutamine

- Disease-related response
  — Dehydration
  — Anterior wall myocardial infarction
  — Chronic heart failure
  — Anemia
  — Shock
    - Sepsis
    - Cardiogenic
    - Hypovolemic
    - Anaphylactic
  — Hyperthyroidism
  — Hypoxia
    - Pulmonary embolism
    - Chronic obstructive pulmonary disease (COPD)

Sinus Tachycardia Assessments

Sinus tachycardia is usually asymptomatic, although the patient may feel palpitations. BUT, remember CO = HR × SV. Therefore, when the heart rate increases; the stroke volume or amount of blood pumped out of the heart with each beat will decrease, resulting in a decreased cardiac output and decreased blood supply to the coronary arteries. The point of elevation in heart rate where the cardiac output may decrease due to reduced ventricular filling time varies from patient to patient based on the individual's physiologic and pathophysiologic state. Unfortunately, the increase in heart rate also increases oxygen demand by the myocardial cells. Chest discomfort or chest pain may result when the cardiac demand for oxygen is unable to be met related to the decreased cardiac output. Sinus tachycardia after a myocardial infarction can point to greater myocardial damage and the initiation of compensatory mechanisms, which may indicate impending chronic heart failure or cardiogenic shock. The decreased ability of the cardiac muscle to contract after a myocardial infarction results in a smaller stroke volume, which is compensated by an elevated heart rate in an attempt to maintain the cardiac output.

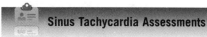

Sinus Tachycardia Assessments

- Usually asymptomatic
- Chest pain
- Syncope/hypotension
- Dyspnea

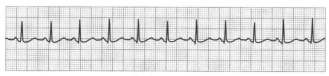

Figure 2-6   Sinus tachycardia.

Sinus Tachycardia Interpretation Criteria

1. Rhythm: regular
2. Rate: 101–180 bpm
3. P wave: upright, uniform, and round in a 1: 1 ratio
4. PRI: between 0.12–0.20 sec
5. QRS I: less than 0.12 sec

Tricks of the Trade

A heart rate greater than 150 bpm initially may be called supraventricular tachycardia (SVT). When the heart beats this fast, the P wave may be obscured into the T wave, making differentiation from other rhythms difficult.

Review Question

What criterion distinguishes sinus tachycardia from NSR?_____

[Heart rate 101–180 bpm]

Sinus Tachycardia Care Measures

When identified as sinus tachycardia, the first step is to identify the effect of the rhythm on the patient's clinical signs and symptoms. If the rhythm is asymptomatic, no treatment is needed. When the rhythm is symptomatic, administer oxygen and obtain IV access, determine and treat the cause such as administer analgesics for pain, administer antipyretics for fever, recommend the dependent position for sexual intercourse, counsel patients on lifestyle choices, administer fluids for dehydration, and provide oxygen for hypoxia. If the rhythm is very rapid causing an obscuring of the P wave into the T wave, the rhythm may need to be treated as a supraventricular tachycardia until the rate can be slowed down enough to determine the underlying rhythm. Vagal maneuvers, adenosine, beta blockers, and calcium channel blockers may be used to slow the heart rate down (AHA, 2005). Recommend following the tachycardia with pulses algorithm suggested by the American Heart Association. See Appendix B.

Sinus Tachycardia Care Measures

- Assess impact of the rhythm on the patient's clinical signs and symptoms
- Treat the cause
- Asymptomatic: no treatment needed.
- Symptomatic
  — Oxygen
  — IV access

— Determine stability

— Vagal maneuvers

— Adenosine

— Beta blockers

— Calcium channel blockers

(2005 American Heart Association Guidelines for Cardiopulmonary Resuscitation and Emergency Cardiovascular Care, Part 2: Ethical Issues. *Circulation*, 2005;112(suppl IV):IV-6-IV-11.)

SINUS DYSRHYTHMIA

Sinus dysrhythmia (SD) is a rhythm initiated by the SA node at an irregular rate. Each beat of this rhythm follows the normal conduction system by traveling from the SA node through the atrial pathway to the AV junctional tissue, down the bundle of His, and out through the Purkinje fibers, leading to atrial followed by ventricular depolarization of the myocardial cells. Two types of sinus dysrhythmia exist: (1) respiratory and (2) nonrespiratory. See Figures 2-7 and 2-8.

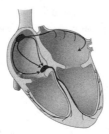

Figure 2-7   Normal conduction pathway in sinus dysrhythmia.

Sinus Dysrhythmia Causes

In respiratory sinus dysrhythmia, the heart rate increases with inspiration and decreases with expiration related to pressure changes within the intrathoracic cavity. In nonrespiratory sinus dysrhythmia, the rhythm is not related to the respiratory cycle.

Sinus Dysrhythmia Causes

- Respiratory
- Nonrespiratory
  - Drug-related response
    - Morphine
    - Digoxin
  - Disease-related response
    - Inferior wall myocardial infarction
    - Increased intracranial pressure

Diversity Impact

A respiratory sinus dysrhythmia is a normal finding in infants and children, but may be observed at other ages. Nonrespiratory sinus dysrhythmia is more likely seen in older adults.

Sinus Dysrhythmia Assessments

No signs and symptoms of the rhythm are seen unless the rhythm is associated with either a sinus bradycardia, known as sinus bradydysrhythmia, or with sinus tachycardia, known as sinus tachydsyrhythmia. When associated with either sinus bradycardia or sinus tachycardia, the signs and symptoms exhibited resemble the assessments found with sinus bradycardia or sinus tachycardia.

Tricks of the Trade

When the patient holds his or her breath for less than 10 seconds, the rhythm becomes regular if the cause of the sinus dysrhythmia is respiratory.

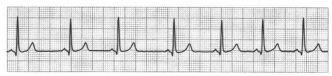

Figure 2-8   Sinus dysrhythmia.

Sinus Dysrhythmia Interpretation Criteria

1. Rhythm: irregular
2. Rate: 60–100 bpm
3. P wave: upright, uniform, and round in a 1:1 ratio
4. PRI: between 0.12– 0.20 sec
5. QRS I: less than 0.12 sec

Review Question

What criterion distinguishes sinus dysrhythmia from NSR? _____

[*Irregular heart rhythm*]

Sinus Dysrhythmia Care Measures

Usually sinus dysrhythmia does not require action, unless associated with symptomatic sinus bradycardia or symptomatic sinus tachycardia. For symptomatic sinus bradydysrhythmia, follow the treatment protocol outlined under sinus bradycardia, and for sinus tachydysrhythmia follow the treatment protocol outlined under sinus tachycardia.

Sinus Dysrhythmia Care Measures

- Assess impact of the rhythm on the patient's clinical signs and symptoms.
- If symptomatic, treat with the appropriate protocol for either sinus tachycardia or sinus bradycardia.

SINOATRIAL ARREST

A lack of automaticity of the SA node can lead to completely dropped complexes of the P, QRS, and T waves. Usually when the SA node does not fire, automaticity of the junctional or ventricular tissue assumes the responsibility for initiating a beat; but if this fails to happen, sinoatrial arrest occurs. When the SA node does fire, each beat of this rhythm follows the normal conduction system by traveling from the SA node through the atrial pathway to the AV junctional tissue, down the bundle of His, and out through the Purkinje fibers, leading to atrial followed by ventricular depolarization of the myocardial cells (Fig. 2-9).

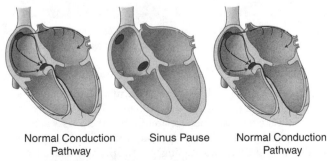

| Normal Conduction Pathway | Sinus Pause | Normal Conduction Pathway |

Figure 2-9   Conduction pathway in sinoatrial arrest.

Sinoatrial Arrest Causes

The main principle behind sinoatrial arrest is a lack of automaticity generated by the SA node triggered by parasympathetic nerve stimulation or ischemia/damage to the SA node area of the heart, which affects the ability of the heart to generate an electrical impulse. Hypoxia or myocardial damage from atherosclerosis to the right coronary artery, which supplies the blood to the SA node area of the heart in 55% of patients, may decrease the SA node's ability to generate an impulse. Drugs that suppress automaticity may lead to sinoatrial arrest.

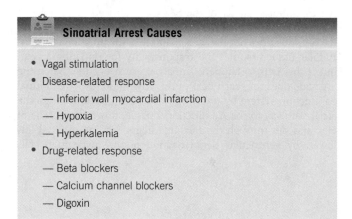

Sinoatrial Arrest Causes

- Vagal stimulation
- Disease-related response
  — Inferior wall myocardial infarction
  — Hypoxia
  — Hyperkalemia
- Drug-related response
  — Beta blockers
  — Calcium channel blockers
  — Digoxin

Sinoatrial Arrest Assessments

The number of dropped complexes determines the seriousness of this rhythm and the effect on the patient's signs and symptoms. The clinical effect becomes apparent when the pauses are more frequent and last for a longer period of time. At that point, the cardiac output decreases, leading to syncope, hypotension, chest pain, and decreased level of consciousness.

Sinoatrial Arrest Assessments

- Usually asymptomatic unless frequent or dropped complexes last for a longer period of time
- Syncope/hypotension
- Chest pain
- Decreased level of consciousness

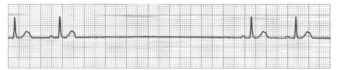

Figure 2-10   Sinoatrial arrest.

Sinoatrial Arrest Interpretation Criteria

1. Rhythm: regular except for dropped complex of P, QRS, and T waves
2. Rate: usually 60–100 bpm, but may vary related to number(s) of dropped complexes
3. P wave: upright, uniform, and round in a 1:1 ratio
4. PRI: between 0.12–0.20 sec
5. QRS I: less than 0.12 sec

Review Question

What criterion distinguishes sinoatrial arrest from NSR? _____

[Occasional completely dropped complexes]

Table 2-1   Practical Comparison of Sinus Rhythms

Distinguishing Features	NSR	SB
Rate (bpm)	60–100	< 60
Rhythm	Regular	Regular/slightly irregular

Sinoatrial Arrest Care Measures

If asymptomatic, no treatment is needed. If mild symptoms exist, the aim is to remove the cause of the rhythm, such as discontinuing beta blocker, calcium channel blocker, or digoxin. For a symptomatic sinoatrial arrest, typically the patient is bradycardic and treatment will follow the symptomatic bradycardia algorithm. Documentation of the rhythm needs to include the underlying rhythm and the length of time of the dropped complexes.

Sinoatrial Arrest Care Measures

- Assess impact of the rhythm on the patient's clinical signs and symptoms
- Symptomatic
  — Oxygen
  — IV access
  — Atropine
  — Transcutaneous or transvenous pacing
- Documentation of the rhythm needs to include the underlying rhythm and the length of the sinoatrial arrest.

ST	SD	SA
101–180	60–100	60–100
Regular	Irregular	Regular except for dropped complexes

PRACTICAL COMPARISON OF SINUS RHYTHMS

Table 2-1 compares the sinus rhythms by rate and rhythm which are the only features that differentiate sinus rhythms from each other. Areas highlighted in red are features of the rhythm which differentiates the rhythm from NSR.

REFERENCE

2005 American Heart Association Guidelines for Cardiopulmonary Resuscitation and Emergency Cardiovascular Care, Part 2: Ethical Issues. *Circulation*, 2005;112(suppl IV):IV-6-IV-11.

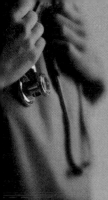

Chapter 3
ATRIAL RHYTHMS

Atrial rhythms are initiated in the atrial tissue of the heart. Atrial rhythms evolve from one of three mechanisms: enhanced automaticity, triggered activity after depolarization, and reentrant mechanisms. Enhanced automaticity is the initiation of impulses in the atrial tissue before the sinoatrial (SA) node is able to generate the impulse. When cells only partially repolarize due to injury, ectopic beats may fire from the tissue repetitively; this is called triggered activity, which is known as afterdepolarizations. Reentrant circuits evolve when impulses are delayed long enough to stimulate another impulse during the repolarization stage. The change in atrial depolarization creates a "funny-looking P wave," meaning P waves that are biphasic (notched), tented, flattened, inverted, or in some way different than the P wave initiated by the patient's SA node. A P wave with an atrial or junctional focus is designated as a P′ wave. For example, a P′ wave may be flattened when it arises from the middle of the right atrium or inverted when the beat is initiated from tissue near the AV junction. Once the beat is conducted through the AV node, the ventricles depolarize and repolarize normally, forming a narrowed QRS. Combinations of dysrhythmias are a common occurrence. One such combination is any atrial dysrhythmia with a bundle branch block. Normally, an atrial rhythm will have a narrow QRS interval. A patient with a bundle branch block may exhibit an atrial dysrhythmia with a wide QRS interval.

PREMATURE ATRIAL CONTRACTIONS (PAC)

Until interpreted, these ectopic beats are frequently and fondly referred to as "funny-looking beats." A premature atrial contraction (PAC) is a solitary beat that originates in the atrial tissue due to enhanced automaticity or a reentry mechanism and occurs every once in a while. A beat created in the atria presents with a P′ wave that is unique in configuration compared to the sinus-originating P waves for the individual patient. From the initiation site, the beat is usually conducted along the normal pathway through the AV junction down the bundle of His and Purkinje fibers (Fig. 3-1). At times, the P′ wave arrives at the AV junction during the refractory period of the previous beat, resulting in a varying shaped P′ wave that is not followed by a QRS complex, called a non-conducted or blocked PAC. When the P′ wave travels at different rates down the bundle branches, the QRS complex becomes wide and is commonly referred to as an aberrantly conducted PAC.

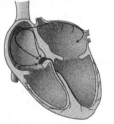
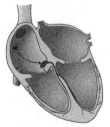

Normal Conduction Pathway

Conduction Pathway in a Premature Atrial Contraction

Figure 3-1   Conduction pathway in premature atrial contraction.

Premature Atrial Contraction Causes

Premature atrial contractions are a common dysrhythmia and may occur normally in response to fear, anxiety, stress, or fatigue. The most prevalent lifestyle activities that cause PACs are nicotine and alcohol. Electrolyte abnormalities that precipitate PACs include hypokalemia and hypomagnesemia. Frequent PACs may be observed in over one-half of all myocardial infarction patients and are often seen in patients with atrial enlargement or chronic heart failure. Chronic obstructive pulmonary disease may be a precipitating factor related to the commonly exhibited signs of atrial enlargement and chronic heart failure associated with this pathophysiology.

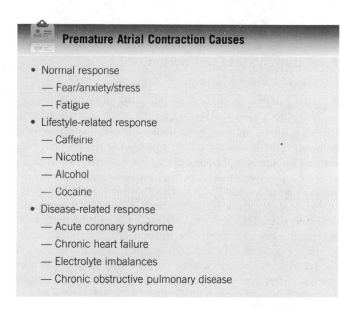

Premature Atrial Contraction Causes

- Normal response
  — Fear/anxiety/stress
  — Fatigue
- Lifestyle-related response
  — Caffeine
  — Nicotine
  — Alcohol
  — Cocaine
- Disease-related response
  — Acute coronary syndrome
  — Chronic heart failure
  — Electrolyte imbalances
  — Chronic obstructive pulmonary disease

Premature Atrial Contraction Assessment

For the most part, patients are asymptomatic except for an irregular pulse. Do not forget to take an apical pulse for 1 minute for all irregular pulses! Palpitations may be experienced, especially if the premature atrial contractions occur often. Extrasystolic beats such as PACs cause a loss of atrial kick for that particular beat, which may lead to syncope and hypotension when the beats recur frequently.

Premature Atrial Contraction Assessment

- Asymptomatic
- Palpitations
- Irregular heart rhythm
- Syncope/hypotension

Premature Atrial Contraction Interpretation Criteria

Because a PAC is a single beat, the underlying ECG rhythm must also be interpreted. An example of documentation of a rhythm might be a normal sinus rhythm with one premature atrial contraction (NSR with a PAC). In a premature atrial contraction, the beat originates in the atrial tissue rather than the sinus node, creating a P′ wave whose shape is distorted or changed from the patient's typical sinus P wave. The P′ wave may be flattened, tented, biphasic, inverted, or obscured within the T wave. The unusually shaped P′ wave is followed by a P′R interval that may be shorter, the same, or longer than the patient's typical P′R interval yet still be between 0.12 and 0.20 seconds. Conduction through the ventricles is normal, creating a narrow QRS complex with an interval of less than 0.12 seconds (Fig. 3-2). If the patient has a concurrent bundle branch block, the QRS may be widened and greater than 0.12 seconds.

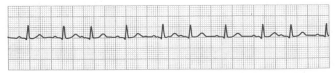

Figure 3-2   Normal sinus rhythm with premature atrial contractions.

Premature Atrial Contraction Interpretation Criteria

1. Rhythm: dependent on underlying rhythm, but usually irregular when PAC occurs
2. Rate: dependent on underlying rhythm's rate, usually 60–100 bpm
3. P' waves: flattened, notched, tented, or inverted P waves
4. P'RI: 0.12–0.20 sec, may vary from sinus beat
5. QRS I: less than 0.12 sec, unless aberrantly conducted or bundle branch block present

Premature atrial contractions present with various characteristics. Recognition and documentation of the characteristics are necessary to treat PACs effectively. Characteristics can be broken into four components: configuration, pattern, frequency in a row, and conduction abnormalities. PACs that originate from the same atrial site will look alike, and are termed monomorphic or unifocal. PACs that originate from different sites in the atrial tissue will appear different in shape and size on the ECG, and are termed polymorphic or multifocal.

The number of PACs per minute can reflect the degree of irritability of the atrial tissue. The greater the number of PACs typically reflects an increase in irritability of the atrial tissue. The frequency of PACs may be documented in two separate ways—by a pattern of beatings or the number of PACs in a row. Premature atrial contractions may occur every other beat intermingled with the patient's underlying rhythm (bigeminy), or every third beat (trigeminy), or every fourth beat (quadrigeminy). PACs may also occur one right after another. Two sequential PACs are called couplets, while three in a row are termed a run. Three or more PACs in a row may be called atrial tachycardia (AT). As the number of PACs per minute increases— as with bigeminy, couplets, runs, and when more than 10 per minute are seen—the rhythm may have more of a clinical impact on the patient related to the potential for decreased cardiac output and the risk for conversion to atrial tachycardia. Premature atrial contractions may precede atrial tachycardia, atrial flutter, or atrial fibrillation (AF) in patients with heart disease.

Two forms of conduction abnormalities are observed with premature atrial contractions: aberrantly conducted PACs and nonconducted or blocked PACs. Aberrantly conducted beats may occur with premature beats and some tachycardias. An aberrantly conducted beat happens when the refractory periods in the two bundle branches are unbalanced, causing the impulse to travel down one bundle branch but delaying conduction through the other bundle branch (Fig. 3-3).

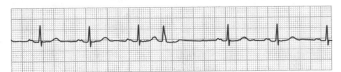

Figure 3-3   Normal sinus rhythm with aberrantly conducted premature atrial contraction.

A nonconducted PAC may also be referred to as a blocked PAC. Premature atrial contractions may be blocked when the extrasystolic beat is initiated too close to the preceding QRS complex, because the AV junction and the bundle branches may still be repolarizing and refractory from the previous beat to respond and conduct the new premature beat (Fig. 3-4). Blocked PACs may be confused with a second-degree heart block known as a Wenckebach block. With blocked PACs, the P′-to-P′ interval is irregular even if the ventricular rate is regular; while the P-to-P interval in a Wenckebach block is regular consistently throughout the rhythm.

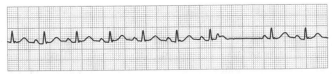

Figure 3-4   Normal sinus rhythm with nonconducted premature atrial contraction.

Characteristics of Premature Atrial Contractions

- Configuration
  - Monomorphic (unifocal): PACs similar in configuration
  - Polymorphic (multifocal): PACs different in configuration
- Pattern
  - Bigeminal: PACs every other beat
  - Trigeminal: PACs every third beat
  - Quadrigeminal: PACs every fourth beat
- Frequency in a row
  - Couplet: 2 PACs in a row
  - Run: 3 or more PACs in a row
- Conduction Abnormalities
  - Aberrantly: early PAC causes difference in conduction time through right and left bundle branches leading to wide QRS complex
  - Nonconducted: early PAC near or in T wave leads to no QRS complex

Review Question

What criteria distinguish this rhythm from NSR?_____

[Flattened, notched, tented, or inverted P' wave. Beat occurs every once in a while.]

Premature Atrial Contraction Care Measures

The first step is to identify the effect of the rhythm on the patient's clinical signs and symptoms. Typically, the rhythm goes undetected or is asymptomatic and requires no treatment. If the rhythm is symptomatic and occurring frequently, then the main focus of treatment is to eradicate the cause. Treatment of the cause is usually centered on reducing fear/anxiety/stress by providing emotional support and medicating with anxiolytics, and instructing patients on lifestyle changes including measures to promote sleep, smoking cessation, methods to reduce caffeine and alcohol intake, and referrals to recreational drug rehabilitation programs. Potassium and magnesium replacements either orally or parenterally may be required to stabilize the myocardial cells and decrease the prevalence of PACs. In patients with underlying heart disease, PACs may be treated with beta blockers or calcium channel blockers.

Premature Atrial Contraction Care Measures

- Assess impact of the rhythm on the patient's clinical signs and symptoms
- Treat the cause
  — Provide emotional support, counseling, and administer anxiolytic medications as needed
  — Instruct patient about sleep-inducing methods and administer sedatives as needed
  — Educate the patient about lifestyle changes
    - Decreasing caffeine intake
    - Smoking cessation
    - Reducing alcohol intake
  — Refer to recreational drug rehabilitation programs
  — Assess electrolyte levels (potassium and magnesium). Adjust dosages for levels to be therapeutic
    - Potassium: normal serum level 4.0–5.0 mEq/L, and 4.3–5 mEq/L in cardiac surgery patients
    - Magnesium: normal serum level 1.8–2.4 mg/dL
  — Treat the cardiac disease-related states
- Administer beta blockers and/or calcium channel blockers

WANDERING ATRIAL PACEMAKER (WAP)

Wandering atrial pacemaker (WAP) is a rhythm that initiates in a variety of supraventricular sites from the SA node to the atrial tissue to the AV junctional area. Due to the varying location of the initiation of the beat between the SA node, atria, and AV junctional tissue, the shape of the P′ wave and length of the P′R interval changes from beat to beat. Impulse conductivity and depolarization through the ventricles is normal, producing a narrow QRS with an interval less than 0.12 seconds. A newer term for this rhythm is multiformed atrial rhythm or atrial bradycardia (Fig. 3-5).

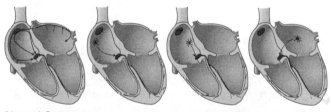

Normal Conduction
Pathway

Conduction Pathway in
Wandering Atrial Pacemaker

Figure 3-5   Conduction pathway in wandering atrial pacemaker.

Wandering Atrial Pacemaker Causes

Wandering atrial pacemaker rhythm may be seen in healthy people during sleep, playing a French horn, or in athletes. Digoxin and organic heart disease can interfere with the automaticity of the heart and the conduction of the impulse through the normal pathway.

Wandering Atrial Pacemaker Causes

- Normal response
  — Athletes
  — Sleep
  — Musicians: French horn players
- Drug-related response
  — Digoxin
- Disease-related response
  — Organic heart disease

Wandering Atrial Pacemaker Assessment

Wandering atrial pacemaker rhythm is usually asymptomatic. With a slow heart rate, the patient could experience some milder symptoms of a decreased cardiac output such as weakness.

Wandering Atrial Pacemaker Interpretation Criteria

Due to the varying sites of automaticity within this rhythm, the P′ waves change in shape and may be upright, uniform, round, flattened, tented, biphasic, or inverted. The P′R interval varies due to the differences in length of time that the impulse takes to travel from varying sites in the SA node, atria, and AV junctional tissue to the AV node. The distinguishing feature between PACs and WAP are the presence of three or more differently shaped P′ waves within the same lead. Multifocal PACs are rare; therefore the shape of the P′ wave for PACs is typically the same within a rhythm strip. See Figure 3-6.

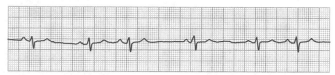

Figure 3-6   Wandering atrial pacemaker.

Wandering Atrial Pacemaker Interpretation Criteria

1. Rhythm: slightly irregular
2. Rate: 60–100 bpm, may be bradycardic
3. P′ waves: shape varies from beat to beat
4. P′RI: 0.12–0.20 sec, but varies from beat to beat
5. QRS I: less than 0.12 sec

Review Question

What criteria distinguish this rhythm from NSR?_____

[*Varying shaped P′ waves and P′R intervals*]

Wandering Atrial Pacemaker Care Measures

The first step is to assess the effect of the rhythm on the patient's clinical state. Because the rhythm resolves spontaneously when the firing of the SA node increases its rate and is typically asymptomatic, no treatment is indicated. An occupational risk of a French horn player can be the conversion to wandering atrial pacemaker when performing. If the cause of the rhythm is due to digoxin, obtaining serum digoxin levels and determining the need to either reduce or discontinue the drug may assist the patient to convert back to normal sinus rhythm. Treatment of heart disease helps to improve perfusion to the heart and may help to maintain cardiac output, preventing the development of signs and symptoms.

Wandering Atrial Pacemaker Care Measures

- Assess impact of the rhythm on the patient's clinical signs and symptoms.
- Treat the cause.
  — Occupational counseling
  — Reduce dose or discontinue digoxin
  — Treat heart disease

ATRIAL TACHYCARDIA (AT)

Atrial tachycardia (AT) is a rhythm originating in the atrial tissue at a rapid rate of 150 to 250 bpm with more than three differently shaped P′ waves in succession. Atrial tachycardia may be classified using several different formats, such as by pathophysiology, anatomy, or origin site of endocardial activation. When classified by pathophysiology, atrial tachycardia is broken into three types: triggered activity, reentry, or enhanced automaticity. Triggered activity is the mechanism behind what is commonly referred to as multifocal atrial tachycardia (MAT). Classification by anatomy is determined by the structural site of impulse initiation, which is either the right or left atrium, although occasionally the rhythm is initiated from the pulmonary vein or superior vena cava. The anatomic location of the rhythm may be determined by assessing the P′ wave in aVL and V_1. An upright P′ wave in aVL usually indicates an impulse site in the right atria, while an upright P′ wave in V_1 usually indicates an impulse site in the left atrium. Endocardial activation site is delineated into focal atrial tachycardia or reentrant atrial tachycardia. Focal atrial tachycardia begins in a localized area of the atria while the reentrant atrial tachycardia usually occurs in areas of structural heart damage or areas of atrial scarring from surgery or heart disease (Okreglicki et al., 2006). The beat originates in the atrial tissue and causes a change in the configuration of the

P' wave. The rate is rapid and may obscure the P' wave in the ST segment or T wave, making the P'R interval indistinguishable. Typically, the ratio of P' waves to QRS complexes is one to one, and the normal conduction pathway in the ventricles elicits a narrow QRS complex. The rhythm may be either regular or irregular depending on the type of atrial tachycardia. In atrial tachycardia with an AV conduction block, the ratio of P' waves to QRS complexes changes to more than one P' wave for every QRS complex (Fig. 3-7).

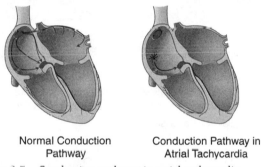

Normal Conduction
Pathway

Conduction Pathway in
Atrial Tachycardia

Figure 3-7   Conduction pathway in atrial tachycardia.

Atrial Tachycardia Causes

Atrial tachycardia may be seen in normal healthy hearts or individuals who are exercising or participating in lifestyle activities such as drinking caffeine or alcohol or using cocaine. These activities increase the catecholamine response and enhance automaticity or cause triggered activity leading to the development of this dysrhythmia. Reentrant tachycardia is more frequently associated with digoxin toxicity. Multifocal atrial tachycardia is often associated with chronic obstructive pulmonary disease, hypoxia, electrolyte imbalances, sympathetic stimulation, and coronary artery disease. Atrial tachycardia that results from scarring or surgeries, particularly in children, is more life threatening.

Atrial Tachycardia Causes

- Normal response
  - Exercise
- Substance-related response
  - Lifestyle
    - Caffeine
    - Alcohol
    - Cocaine
  - Drugs
    - Digoxin
    - Albuterol
    - Theophylline
- Disease-related response
  - Congenital heart disease surgeries: Fontan procedure
  - Valvular heart disease
  - Hypoxia
  - Chronic heart failure
  - Chronic obstructive pulmonary disease

Atrial Tachycardia Assessment

Remember cardiac output equals heart rate multiplied by stroke volume. When the heart rate speeds up, the stroke volume decreases related to reduced time for ventricular filling, resulting in a lower cardiac output. The shortened diastole may cause decreased coronary artery perfusion at a time when the oxygen consumption from the rapid heart rate has increased. When the rhythm does not last long, the patient may be asymptomatic or have mild symptoms of fatigue and weakness. When the rhythm is prolonged, the patient decompensates and exhibits signs of diminished cardiac output including chest pain, syncope/hypotension, and dyspnea. The end product can extend from angina to myocardial infarction to heart failure. Multifocal atrial tachycardia may evolve into atrial fibrillation.

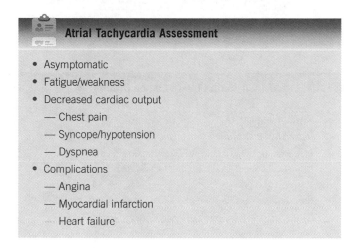

Atrial Tachycardia Assessment

- Asymptomatic
- Fatigue/weakness
- Decreased cardiac output
  — Chest pain
  — Syncope/hypotension
  — Dyspnea
- Complications
  — Angina
  — Myocardial infarction
  — Heart failure

Atrial Tachycardia Interpretation Criteria

Atrial tachycardia is most commonly seen in a one P′ wave to one QRS complex ratio at a rapid regular rate of 150 to 250 bpm. At least three variously shaped P′ waves need to be observed in the ECG strip for the interpretation of atrial tachycardia to be made. The P′ wave is typically upright, but may be obscured within the ST segment or T wave. When the P′ wave is obscured, it becomes difficult to identify a difference in the P′ wave and the P′R interval becomes perhaps impossible to measure. The anatomic location of the rhythm may be determined by assessing the P′ wave in aVL and V_1. An upright P′ wave in aVL usually indicates an impulse site in the right atria, while an upright P′ wave in V_1 usually indicates an impulse site in the left atrium. In digoxin toxicity, the classic ECG tracing is atrial tachycardia with an AV conduction block portrayed by more than one P′ wave per QRS (Fig. 3-8).

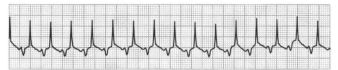

Figure 3-8   Atrial tachycardia.

Atrial Tachycardia Interpretation Criteria

1. Rhythm: regular
2. Rate: 150–250 bpm
3. P′ waves: upright, round, vary in shape from sinus P wave, may be obscured in ST segment or T wave
4. P′RI: 0.12–0.20 sec, varies from sinus beats; may be indistinguishable when buried in T wave
5. QRS I: usually less than 0.12 sec

Review Question

What criteria distinguish atrial tachycardia from NSR?_____

[Varying shaped P′ waves and P′R intervals with heart rate of 150 to 250 bpm]

Multifocal atrial tachycardia (MAT) may be inadvertently diagnosed as atrial fibrillation related to the irregularity of the rhythm. The classic characteristics of MAT are an irregular rhythm with three or more differently configured P′ waves at a rate of 100 to 200 bpm, with the key to distinguishing the rhythm from atrial fibrillation as a flat isoelectric line between the easily identified P′ waves. A rate of less than 100 bpm classifies MAT as a wandering atrial pacemaker (Fig. 3-9).

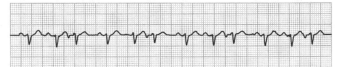

Figure 3-9   Multifocal atrial tachycardia.

Multifocal Atrial Tachycardia Interpretation Criteria

1. Rhythm: irregular for atria and ventricles
2. Rate: 100 200 bpm
3. P' waves: shape varies from beat to beat
4. P'RI: usually 0.12–0.20 sec, but varies from beat to beat
5. QRS I: usually less than 0.12 sec

Atrial Tachycardia Care Measures

The first step is to determine the effect of the atrial tachycardia on the patient's clinical symptomatology and then to consider the possible causes of the rhythm in that individual patient. Due to the rapidity of the rhythm, interpretation may be difficult, and the rhythm may be called a supraventricular tachycardia and treated with the Tachycardia with Pulses algorithm suggested by the American Heart Association (see Appendix B). Once the rhythm has been slowed, the actual site of the dysrhythmia may be determined, allowing for more appropriate actions. For patients who experience atrial tachycardia related to lifestyle choices, educational and support programs are needed to alter behaviors. Serum digoxin levels need to be monitored for any patient receiving digoxin to prevent the development of this rhythm from digoxin toxicity. Children with congenital heart defects, particularly post-operative Fontan surgery, are the most likely candidates for instability and requiring synchronized cardioversion. Multifocal atrial tachycardia rarely needs to be treated. When the Tachycardia with Pulses algorithm is applied to the MAT patient, no response is seen when the patient receives carotid massage. The treatment for MAT is usually administering oxygen and caring for the patient's COPD, which may indicate albuterol inhalers. Since albuterol may have caused this rhythm, careful consideration of the individual patient and his or her response to albuterol and their physical status needs to occur. This may be a *Catch 22*! Recent research has led to the creation of an algorithm to identify the P′ wave site of focal atrial tachycardia, which opens the door for more accurate ECG interpretation and identification of the area for radiofrequency ablation (Kistler et al., 2006). Catheter ablation may be used to treat focal atrial tachycardias.

Atrial Tachycardia Care Measures

- Assess impact of the rhythm on the patient's clinical signs and symptoms
- Determine stability of the patient
- Administer oxygen and obtain IV access

Stable	**Unstable**
• Perform vagal maneuvers	• Perform synchronized cardioversion
• Administration of adenosine	
• Administration of beta blockers and/or calcium channel blockers	
• Prevent/treat the underlying cause	

- Prevent/treat the underlying cause
  — Educate the patient about lifestyle changes
    ▪ Counseling, stress reduction techniques, and anxiolytic agents
    ▪ Sleep-inducing methods and hypnotics
    ▪ Decreasing caffeine intake
  — Refer to recreational drug rehabilitation programs
- Radiofrequency catheter ablation

(2005 American Heart Association Guidelines for Cardiopulmonary Resuscitation and Emergency Cardiovascular Care, Part 2: Ethical Issues. *Circulation*, 2005;112(suppl IV):IV-6-IV-11.)

ATRIAL FLUTTER (A FLUTTER)

Atrial flutter initiates in a single location of the atria causing rapid depolarization of the atrial tissue. Usually, atrial flutter has a single reentrant circuit with a counterclockwise circular activation near the tricuspid valve in the right atrium, creating an atrial rate of 240 to 450 bpm. An AV block limits the number of impulses reaching the ventricles, creating a ventricular rate of 60 to 180 bpm. Once the beat reaches the bundle branches, the impulse travels normally through bundle of His and the Purkinje fibers, usually creating a narrow QRS. Atrial flutter has been further delineated into type I and type II, which vary based on several characteristics such as anatomic location of impulse site, cause of rhythm, and atrial rate. Due to a lack of understanding about the entire mechanism of this rhythm, traditional classification is still used to describe atrial flutter based upon its classic sawtooth pattern of atrial activity seen on the ECG (Fig. 3-10).

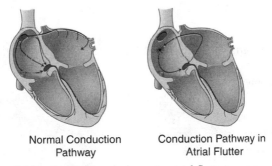

Normal Conduction
Pathway

Conduction Pathway in
Atrial Flutter

Figure 3-10   Conduction pathway in atrial flutter.

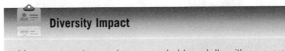

Diversity Impact

More commonly seen in men and older adults with an average age of 64 years. Not frequently seen in children unless they have congential heart defects. Pregnant women with dysrhythmias or heart disease have increased risk for themselves and their fetus.

Atrial Flutter Causes

Initiation of the rhythm may occur after a premature atrial contraction as a result of enhanced automaticity or as a single-circuit reentry mechanism. Enhanced automaticity may occur from irritating substances or sympathetic stimulation such as fear, anxiety, stress, and lifestyle substances including caffeine, alcohol, and nicotine. Type I atrial flutter is more commonly seen in patients with compromised left ventricular function such as myocardial infarction, chronic heart failure, and chronic obstructive pulmonary disease. Fluid overload may precipitate this rhythm from elevated right atrial pressure and hypertrophy. Most recently, diabetes mellitus has been linked to the development of atrial flutter (Movahed et al., 2005). Type II atrial flutter is more apt to be seen in patients after cardiac surgery evolving near the cardiac surgical scar or the mitral valve.

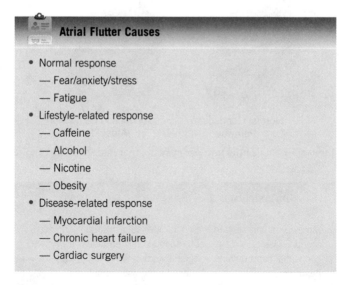

Atrial Flutter Causes

- Normal response
  — Fear/anxiety/stress
  — Fatigue
- Lifestyle-related response
  — Caffeine
  — Alcohol
  — Nicotine
  — Obesity
- Disease-related response
  — Myocardial infarction
  — Chronic heart failure
  — Cardiac surgery

- ■ Adult—coronary artery bypass graft/valve replacements
- ■ Pediatrics—Fontan/Senning/Mustard procedures
— Hyperthyroidism
— Chronic obstructive pulmonary disease (COPD)

Atrial Flutter Assessment

Although atrial flutter may be asymptomatic, patients generally exhibit signs and symptoms of decreased cardiac output. Palpitations are commonly felt by patients. Toleration of the rhythm by the patient is mostly determined by the ventricular response rate and degree of AV conduction block. A higher ventricular response rate and lower amount of AV block leads to increased symptoms due to lower ventricular filling times and the loss of atrial kick. The symptoms are reflective of a decreased cardiac output such as chest pain from decreased coronary artery perfusion, syncope and hypotension from decreased forward blood flow, and dyspnea from blood accumulation leading to pulmonary congestion.

 Atrial Flutter Assessment

- Asymptomatic
- Palpitations/fatigue
- Chest pain
- Syncope/hypotension
- Dyspnea

Atrial Flutter Interpretation Criteria

Atrial flutter is most easily interpreted in leads II, III, aVF, and V_1. The classic characteristic of atrial flutter is a sawtooth pattern of atrial waves known as flutter waves, not P waves. Type I atrial flutter has atrial rates of 240 to 340 bpm and represents the hallmark picture of atrial flutter. Type II atrial flutter has atrial rates of 341 to 450 bpm and due to the rapidity of the rhythm is not as well representative of the hallmark picture of atrial flutter. If the rhythm has a rapid ventricular response rate, the sawtooth atrial pattern may be obscured. Performing vagal maneuvers can slow the ventricular response rate to the point that the sawtooth pattern exhibits itself. The atrial rate is regular, but due to varying conduction ratios through the AV node the ventricular rate may vary between 60 and 180 bpm, usually no more than 150 bpm. The block could occur at a constant ratio of 2:1, 3:1, or 4:1, making the ventricular rhythm regular; or the conduction ratio may vary from beat to beat, making the ventricular rhythm irregular. Once the beat passes through the AV node, the ventricular depolarization process is usually normal, presenting a narrow QRS of less than 0.12 seconds. When the ventricular rate is greater than 100 bpm, the rhythm is considered to be uncontrolled with a rapid ventricular response (RVR). Documentation of the rhythm denotes the conduction ratio, presence of RVR, as well as the rhythm state such as "A-flutter with RVR at a 2:1 conduction ratio" (Fig 3-11).

Tricks of the Trade

Turning the strip upside down will look very similar to right side up, which helps in interpretation of this rhythm.

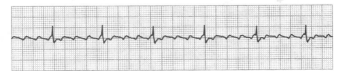

Figure 3-11   Atrial flutter.

Atrial Flutter Interpretation Criteria

1. Rhythm:
   A. Atrial: regular
   B. Ventricular: regular or irregular depending on AV conduction ratio
2. Rate:
   A. Atrial: 240–450 bpm
   B. Ventricular: varies usually between 60–180 bpm
3. P waves: flutter waves with sawtooth appearance
4. PRI: none
5. QRS I: less than 0.12 sec

Review Question

What criteria distinguish this rhythm from NSR?_____

[Sawtooth flutter waves with atrial rate 240–450 bpm]

Atrial Flutter Care Measures

Typically, atrial flutter is a temporary rhythm, and patients will either convert back to normal sinus rhythm or progress into atrial fibrillation. As with most rhythms, determining the effect of the rhythm on the patient's medical stability is critical to deciding on the treatment regimen. Stability of the patient is decided based on the level of acuity of the symptoms. Unstable patients exhibit hypotension, chest pain, and change in level of consciousness and usually have pulses greater than 150 bpm. Three main routes of atrial flutter therapy exist today: electrical cardioversion, anti-dysrhythmic agents, and catheter ablation. If the rhythm is uncontrolled with a rapid ventricular response, following the Tachycardia with Pulses algorithm suggested by the American Heart Association is recommended (see Appendix B). A 12-lead ECG is recommended to differentiate atrial flutter from other supraventricular rhythms. Treatment for an unstable patient with atrial flutter is to administer synchronized cardioversion. To avoid and/or decrease the risk of a cerebrovascular accident, a transesophageal echocardiogram may be helpful to determine the presence of thrombus in the left atrium. Cardioversion is held if the patient has been in atrial flutter for an unidentified period of time or longer than 48 hours until the patient has been anti-coagulated. If the rhythm is stable with a narrow QRS, vagal maneuvers and adenosine may help to diagnose the rapid rhythm as atrial flutter by temporarily slowing the conduction through the AV node. Beta blockers and diltiazem may be used to control rate by slowing conduction via the AV node. Other anti-dysrhythmics that may be used to convert atrial flutter to normal sinus rhythm are ibutilide and dofetilide, which prolong the action potential in depolarization. Digoxin may also be used to control ventricular rate by slowing down AV conduction, particularly with fetal atrial flutter. Atrial pacing has some use immediately after open heart surgery when pacing wires are still available. Catheter ablation is used for patients with symptoms that affect their quality of life (Boyer & Koplan, 2005) and is more effective on type I atrial flutter. Cauterization of the atrial sites responsible for the rhythm is zapped through catheters directed at the sites. Scar tissue develops, which prevents the circuitous reentrant activity and enhanced automaticity of the troubled atrial sites.

Atrial Flutter Care Measures

- Assess impact of the rhythm on the patient's clinical signs and symptoms
- Treat causes
- Obtain IV access

Stable
- Obtain 12-lead ECG

Regular Rhythm
- If QRS narrow, perform vagal maneuvers
- If rhythm does not convert, administer adenosine at 6 mg. May repeat adenosine dosing at 12 mg two times
- Repeat adenosine and/or try beta blockers or diltiazem

Irregular Rhythm
- Obtain cardiology consult
- Administer beta blockers or diltiazem

Unstable
- Prepare and deliver synchronized cardioversion

(2005 American Heart Association Guidelines for Cardiopulmonary Resuscitation and Emergency Cardiovascular Care, Part 2: Ethical Issues. *Circulation*, 2005;112(suppl IV): IV-6-IV-11.)

ATRIAL FIBRILLATION (AF)

Atrial fibrillation (AF) is a rhythm initiated in multiple sites of the atria, typically in the left atrium. Enhanced automaticity and reentrant circuit pathways create a rapid firing of impulses. Between 350 and 650 impulses are generated each minute, which creates a chaotic firing of atrial impulses being transmitted to the AV node. Due to the rapidity and number of impulses being fired, the atria become a quivering mass without ability to functionally contract blood forcefully into the ventricles. Depolarizations from one impulse only spread in the atria a short distance, and many do not reach the AV node. Impulses generated near the AV node are conducted through the AV node in a sporadic fashion, which creates an irregular ventricular rhythm. The impulse travels normally through the bundle of His and Purkinje fibers. The ECG will show a chaotic isoelectric line without P waves or PR interval and typically a narrow QRS complex in a grossly irregular pattern (Fig. 3-12). Typically, atrial fibrillation will first present itself as an uncontrolled rhythm with a rapid ventricular response and heart rate of 160 to 180 bpm. The atrial fibrillation is controlled when the heart rate is 60 to 100 bpm. Atrial fibrillation is classified by the three Ps based on the patient's ability to convert to normal sinus rhythm: paroxysmal, persistent, and permanent. Paroxysmal atrial fibrillation occurs when the rhythm starts and stops spontaneously. Persistent atrial fibrillation occurs when electrical shock and/or drug therapy is needed to convert the patient back to NSR. Permanent atrial fibrillation occurs when attempts to cardiovert back to NSR fail after the use of drugs or electrical shock, or if conversion to NSR is not maintained. Atrial fibrillation is the most common dysrhythmia, accounting for over one-third of the hospitalizations for dysrhythmias and greater than 1.5 billion U.S. health dollars per year.

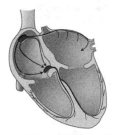
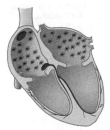

Normal Conduction   Conduction Pathway in
Pathway   Atrial Fibrillation

Figure 3-12   Conduction pathway in atrial fibrillation.

Diversity Impact

More commonly seen in men and older adults

Atrial Fibrillation Causes

Atrial fibrillation may occur in healthy individuals or as a disease-related response. When atrial fibrillation is seen in healthy people, the rhythm is called lone atrial fibrillation due to an idiopathic cause. Increased sympathetic or parasympathetic tone may cause this rhythm, in response to caffeine, nicotine, alcohol, fear/anxiety/stress, and vomiting. Many times, atrial fibrillation is due to atrial dilation, which elevates the pressure in the atria (mitral valve disorders, chronic heart failure, rheumatic heart disease). Approximately one-third of patients after cardiac or pulmonary surgery experience this rhythm.

Atrial Fibrillation Causes

- Healthy individuals
- Lifestyle-related response
  — Caffeine
  — Alcohol
  — Nicotine
  — Exercise
  — Fear/anxiety/stress
- Disease-related response
  — Rheumatic heart disease
  — Chronic heart failure
  — Coronary artery disease/myocardial infarction
  — Cardiac surgery
  — Mitral valve stenosis/regurgitation

Atrial Fibrillation Assessment

Generally, atrial fibrillation is better tolerated than atrial flutter. Because the ventricular rhythm is grossly irregular, each patient will present with an irregular pulse. A pulse deficit may be found when the apical and radial pulses taken simultaneously are unequal. The slower radial pulse is produced due to a lack of ventricular filling and weaker myocardial contractions. A decreased cardiac output with its associated signs and symptoms occurs related to a loss of atrial kick and decreased ventricular filling. Two main complications of atrial fibrillation are (1) chronic heart failure due to the blood pooling in the atria from the lack of atrial contraction and inability of the atria to propel the blood into the ventricles; and (2) emboli due to pooling of the blood in the atria causing clots to form, which then travel, leading to strokes, myocardial infarctions, and pulmonary emboli.

Atrial Fibrillation Assessment

- Irregular pulse
- Pulse deficit
- Decreased cardiac output
  - Fatigue
  - Dyspnea
  - Syncope/hypotension
  - Chest pain
- Chronic heart failure
- Emboli
  - Cerebrovascular accident (stroke)
  - Myocardial infarction
  - Pulmonary embolus

Atrial Fibrillation Interpretation Criteria

The rhythm is usually best seen in lead II. P waves are not seen; instead the atrial activity is depicted by fibrillatory waves. A larger chaotic fibrillatory baseline is called coarse atrial fibrillation, while a smoother baseline between the R-R waves is named fine atrial fibrillation. Without P waves, the PRI is not able to be determined. The QRS is narrow and less than 0.12 seconds usually due to normal ventricular depolarization. A key to identifying this rhythm is the grossly irregular R-R rhythm. If the ventricular rate is less than 100 bpm, the rate is considered to be controlled (Fig. 3-13).

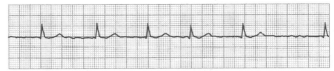

Figure 3-13   Controlled atrial fibrillation.

If the ventricular rate is rapid, the T waves may not be able to be distinguished. When the ventricular rate is greater than 100 bpm, the rhythm is considered to be uncontrolled with a rapid ventricular response (RVR). Documentation of the rhythm denotes the presence of RVR as well as the rhythm state such as "AF with RVR" (Fig. 3-14).

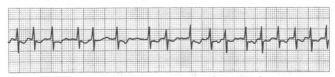

Figure 3-14   Atrial fibrillation with rapid ventricular response.

Atrial Fibrillation Interpretation Criteria

1. Rhythm:
   A. Atrial: chaotic baseline
   B. Ventricular: grossly irregular
2. Rate:
   A. Atrial: 350–650 bpm, unable to be determined
   B. Ventricular:
      i. Controlled: 60–100 bpm
      ii. Uncontrolled: 101–200 bpm
3. P waves: none seen
4. PRI: none
5. QRS I: less than 0.12 sec

Review Question

What criteria distinguish this rhythm from NSR?_____

[Chaotic wavy baseline with grossly irregular ventricular
rhythm. Heart rate: 60 to 200 bpm.]

Atrial Fibrillation Care Measures

The first step is to assess the effects of the rhythm on the patient's
clinical signs and symptoms. A patient with a rapid ventricular
response would be expected to be more symptomatic.
Hemodynamic instability is based on the presence of hypotension,
chest pain, and changes in mental status. The second step is to
determine the length of time that the patient has been experiencing the rhythm. When a patient has been in atrial fibrillation for
more than 48 hours or an indeterminate amount of time, a risk for
emboli exists if the patient is converted immediately back to normal sinus rhythm. For unstable patients with RVR who have

experienced the rhythm for less than 48 hours, elective synchronized cardioversion is planned to attempt to convert the patient back
into NSR. For synchronized cardioversion, obtain informed con-
sent and sedate prior to performing procedure. A transesophageal
echocardiogram (TEE) is frequently performed before cardioversion
to determine the presence of thrombus in the heart. Anti-coagulation
therapy is typically needed prior to cardioversion for patients with
an indeterminate amount of time or more than 48 hours of main-
tenance of atrial fibrillation. Following the Tachycardia with Pulses
algorithm suggested by the American Heart Association is recommended (Appendix B). For the patient with hemodynamic stability,
beta blockers (metoprolol) or calcium channel blockers (diltiazem)
may be administered intravenously for rate control. Occasionally,
the slowing of the ventricular response rate may actually lead to
conversion to normal sinus rhythm. Due to the risk for clot formation, ACC/AHA/ESC recommends guidelines for assessment of
stroke risk and prevention with use of anti-coagulant in patients
with atrial fibrillation (Table 3-1).

For many years a quiet controversy has existed related to what
is the main goal of treatment of atrial fibrillation: rate control or
rhythm control (see the Evidenced-Based Practice box later in the
chapter). A recent study in the *New England Journal of Medicine*
found no significant difference in mortality rates for patients with
chronic heart failure and atrial fibrillation between a rhythm control
strategy and a rate control strategy treatment plan (Roy et al., 2008).
This study is only one of a long line of investigations on this subject
such as the AFFIRM (Atrial Fibrillation Follow-up Investigation
of Rhythm Management), RACE (Rate Control versus Electrical
Cardioversion for persistent atrial fibrillation), STAF (Strategies of
Treatment of Atrial Fibrillation), and PIAF (Pharmacologic
Intervention in Atrial Fibrillation) (Carlsson et al., 2003; Cooper
et al., 2004; Gronefeld et al., 2003; Van Gelder et al., 2002). The controversy continues, as no significant difference has been found
between rate and rhythm control strategies. Radiofrequency catheter
ablation is recommended for patients when neither cardioversion
nor drug therapy are effective. For chronic atrial fibrillation, oral
administration of propafenone, dofetilide, and amiodarone are
possible agents to use to convert to NSR.

Table 3-1   Antithrombotic Therapy for Patients with Atrial Fibrillation

Risk Category	Recommended Therapy
No risk factors	Aspirin, 81–325 mg daily
One moderate-risk factor	Aspirin, 81–325 mg daily, or warfarin (INR 2.0–3.0 m, target 2.5)
Any high-risk factor or more than one moderate-risk factor	Warfarin (INR 2.0–3.0, target 2.5)[a]

Less Validated or Weaker Risk Factors	Moderate-Risk Factors	High-Risk Factors
Female gender	Age greater than or equal to 75 y	Previous stroke, TIA, or embolism
Age 65–74 y	Hypertension	Mitral stenosis
Coronary artery disease	Heart Failure	Prosthetic heart valve[a]
Thyrotoxicosis	LV ejection fraction 35% or less	
	Diabetes mellitus	

[a]If mechanical valve, target international normalized ratio (INR) greater than 2.5.

LV, left ventricular; TIA, transient ischemic attack.

Reprinted from American College/American Heart Association Task Force and the European Society of Cardiology Committee for Practice Guidelines, 48, Fuster V, Ryden LE, Cannom DS, et al., ACC/AHA/ESC 2006 guidelines for the management of patients with atrial fibrillation—executive summary: a report of the American College/American Heart Association Task Force and the European Society of Cardiology Committee for Practice Guidelines (writing committee to revise the 2001 guidelines for the management of patients with atrial fribrillation), 877, 2006 with permission form Elsevier.

Atrial Fibrillation Care Measures

- Assess impact of the rhythm on the patient's clinical signs and symptoms
- Provide oxygen and obtain IV access
- Treat causes

Hemodynamic Stability
- Obtain cardiology consult
- Administer beta blockers or diltiazem

- Evaluate need for anti-coagulation
- Administer propafenone, dofetilide, or amiodarone
- Radiofrequency catheter ablation

Hemodynamic Instability
- Prepare and deliver synchronized cardioversion
- Obtain TEE
- Obtain cardioversion procedure permission
- Consider need for anti-coagulation

(2005 American Heart Association Guidelines for Cardiopulmonary Resuscitation and Emergency Cardiovascular Care, Part 2: Ethical Issues. *Circulation*, 2005;112(suppl IV):IV-6-IV-11.)

Evidenced-Based Practice

The purpose of the study was to determine the outcome on mortality rates for rhythm versus rate control therapy in patient with atrial fibrillation and heart failure. Using multiple clinical sites, the investigators randomly assigned 1376 participants to treatments to either maintain NSR or to control the ventricular rate. The rhythm control groups received amiodarone and more than one treatment of cardioversion, while the rate control group received beta blockers and digoxin to obtain a specific heart rate target. The dependent variable was death by cardiovascular causes, death due to other causes, deteriorating chronic heart failure, stroke, and hospitalizations. Data indicate a similar effect on mortality rates from rhythm and rate control strategies in treatment of atrial fibrillation in patients with chronic heart failure (Roy et al., 2008).

PRACTICAL COMPARISON OF ATRIAL RHYTHMS

Table 3-2 compares the atrial rhythms by rate, rhythm, P waves, and PR intervals which are the features that differentiate atrial rhythms from each other. Areas highlighted in red are features of the rhythm which differentiates the rhythm from Normal Sinus Rhythm.

Table 3-2   Practical Comparison of Atrial Rhythms

Distinguishing Features	NSR	PAC	WAP
Rhythm	Regular	Irregular when beat occurs	Slightly irregular
Rate (bpm)	60–100	Usually 60–100	60–100, bradycardic
P wave	Upright, uniform, & round	Flattened, notched, tented, or inverted	Shape varies beat to beat
PRI	0.12–0.20 sec	0.12–0.20 sec	0.12–0.20 sec, varies beat to beat

NSR, normal sinus rhythm; PAC, premature atrial contraction; WAP, wandering atrial pacemaker; AT, atrial tachycardia; A-flutter, atrial flutter; AF, atrial fibrillation.

AT	A-Flutter	AF
Regular	Atrial: regular Ventricular: regular or irregular	Atrial chaotic baseline Ventricular grossly irregular
150–250	Atrial: 240–450 Ventricular: 60–180	Atrial: unable to be determined Ventricular: 60–200
Varied shape, may be obscured into T wave	Flutter waves with sawtooth appearance	None
Usually 0.12–0.20	None	None

REFERENCES

Boyer M, Koplan BA. Atrial flutter. *Circulation*. 2005. Retrieved on September 29, 2008 from http://circ.ahajournals.org/cgi/content/full/112/22/e334.

Carlsson J, Miketic S, Windeler J, et al. Randomized trial of rate-control versus rhythm-control in persistent atrial fibrillation: the Strategies of Treatment of Atrial Fibrillation (STAF) study. *J Am Coll Cardiol.* 2003;41:1690–1696.

Cooper HA, Bloomfield DA, Bush DE, et al. Relation between achieved heart rate and outcomes in patients with atrial fibrillation. *Am J Cardiol.* 2004;93:1247–1253.

2005 American Heart Association Guidelines for Cardiopulmonary Resuscitation and Emergency Cardiovascular Care, Part 2: Ethical Issues. *Circulation,* 2005;112(suppl IV):IV-6-IV-11.

Fuster V, Ryden LE, Cannom DS, et al. ACC/AHA/ESC 2006 guidelines for the management of patients with atrial fibrillation— executive summary: a report of the American College of Cardiology American Heart Association Task Force and the European Society of Cardiology Committee for Practice Guidelines (writing committee to revise the 2001 guidelines for the management of patients with atrial fribrillation). *J Am Coll Cardiol.* 2006;48:854–906.

Gronefeld GC, Lilienthal J, Kuck KH, et al. Impact of rate versus rhythm control on quality of life in patients with persistent atrial fibrillation: results from a prospective randomized study. *Eur Heart J.* 2003;24:1430–1436.

Kistler PM, Roberts-Thomson KC, Haqqani HM, et al. P-wave morphology in focal atrial tachycardia: development of an algorithm to predict the anatomic site of origin. *J Am Coll Cardiol.* 2006;48: 1010–1017.

Movahed MR, Hashemzadeh M, Jamal MM. Diabetes mellitus is a strong, independent risk for atrial fibrillation and flutter in addition to other cardiovascular disease. *Int J Cardiol.* 2005;105:315–318.

Okreglicki A, Hongsheng MG, Rosero S, et al. Atrial tachycardia. 2006. Retrieved on November 4, 2008 from http://www.emedicine.com/Med/topic188.htm.

Roy D, Talajic RD, Nattel S, et al. Rhythm control versusrate control for atrial fibrillation and heart failure. *N Engl J Med.* 2008; 358:2667–2677.

Van Gelder IC, Hagens VE, Bosker HA, et al. A comparison of rate control and rhythm control in patients with recurrent persistent atrial fibrillation. *N Engl J Med.* 2002;347:1834–1840.

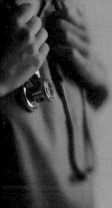

Chapter 4

JUNCTIONAL RHYTHMS

Junctional rhythms are initiated in the junctional tissue of the heart. Junctional tissue is located around the AV node and includes the bundle of His before it separates into the right and left branches in the upper section of the interventricular septum. Junctional tissue has automaticity that may initiate beats at an inherent rate of 40 to 60 bpm. Junctional rhythms occur due to failure of the SA node to fire (sinoatrial arrest), initiation of impulses in the SA node less than 40 bpm (sinus bradycardia), or blockage of conduction of a beat originating in the SA node (sinus block). Each junctional beat flows simultaneously in two directions: (1) retrograde depolarization occurs as the impulse flows backward through the atria, forming an inverted P wave with a shortened PR interval, a missing P wave, or an inverted P wave after the QRS, which may change the appearance of the QRS; and (2) a normal or antegrade depolarization process through the ventricles eliciting a typical QRS complex and QRS interval of 0.06 to 0.12 seconds.

 Tricks of the Trade

Inverted P waves will be seen in leads II, III, and aVF; yet may still be upright in leads I and aVR.

PREMATURE JUNCTIONAL CONTRACTIONS (PJC)

Until interpreted, these ectopic beats are frequently and fondly referred to as "funny-looking beats." A premature junctional contraction (PJC) is a beat that originates in the junctional tissue either from irritability or as a "fail-safe" mechanism when the SA node fails to initiate the beat or the beat is blocked in these higher pacemaker sites. If the PJC beat occurs before expected based on the patient's underlying rhythm with a short R-R interval between the preceding beat and the early PJC beat, the cause is attributable to irritability. When the PJC beat occurs later than expected based on the patient's underlying rhythm with a longer R-R interval between the preceding beat and the late PJC beat, the cause is attributable to a "fail-safe" mechanism due to a lack of performance by the SA node. Fail-safe beats are occasionally referred to as junctional escape beats. When a junctional contraction is a solitary beat surrounded by other sinus beats, the differentiation between a premature beat and an escape beat becomes easy to view and important to understand when considering treatment. Despite the importance of the differentiation between prematurity and escape beats, in clinical practice all solitary junctional beats are usually referred to as PJCs. Each junctional beat flows simultaneously in two directions: (1) retrograde depolarization occurs as the impulse flows backward through the atria forming an inverted P wave with a shortened PR interval, a missing P wave, or an inverted P wave after the QRS, which may change the appearance of the QRS; and (2) a normal or antegrade depolarization process through the ventricles eliciting a typical QRS complex and QRS interval of 0.06 to 0.12 seconds. A P wave in a junctional rhythm is designated as a P' regardless of its configuration (Fig. 4-1).

Premature Junctional Contraction Causes

PJCs may occur in healthy people without an identified cause. The most common cause of PJCs is an elevated digoxin level greater than 2.5 ng/mL. Therapeutic digoxin levels are 0.9 to 1.5 ng/mL, but toxic levels of greater than 1.5 ng/mL are regularly seen, particularly in patients taking loop or thiazide diuretics. Digoxin, quinidine, and

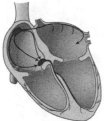 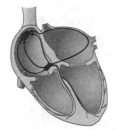

Normal Conduction
Pathway

Conduction Pathway in Premature
Junctional Contraction

Figure 4-1   Conduction pathway in premature junctional
contractions.

procainamide cause PJCs by suppressing the initiation of the beat at
the SA node while methamphetamine causes PJCs due to irritability
of the AV junctional tissue. The disease-related responses occur due
to irritability or actual damage to the heart tissue, typically in the
location of the SA node or the AV junctional tissue.

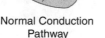

Premature Junctional Contraction Causes

- Fatigue
- Substance-related response
  — Lifestyle-related response
    - Caffeine
    - Tobacco
    - Cocaine
  — Drug-related response
    - Digoxin, levels greater than 2.5 ng/mL (frequent
      cause)
    - Quinidine
    - Beta blockers
    - Calcium channel blockers
    - Methamphetamine

- Disease-related response
  — Inferior wall myocardial infarction
  — Rheumatic heart disease
  — Inflammation after cardiac surgery
  — Chronic heart failure
  — Electrolyte disturbances
    ▪ Hypokalemia
    ▪ Hypomagnesemia

Premature Junctional Contraction Assessment

Infrequent PJCs of less than 10 per minute are considered to be clinically insignificant. An irregular pulse is generated related to the early or late response of the junctional tissue to either irritability of the junctional tissue or lack of initiation of impulse by the SA node. Palpitations, a sensing of one's heart beating within the chest, may be felt particularly with an increased frequency of PJCs per minute. As the number of PJCs per minute increase, the cardiac output may decrease, causing hypotension.

Premature Junctional Contraction Assessment

- Usually clinically insignificant
- Irregular pulse
- Palpitations
- Decreased cardiac output
  — Dizziness
  — Hypotension

Premature Junctional Contraction Interpretation Criteria

Because a PJC is a single beat, the underlying ECG rhythm must also be interpreted. An example of documentation of a rhythm might be sinus bradycardia with one premature junctional contraction (SB with a PJC). Differentiation between premature atrial contractions (PAC) with inverted P′ waves and PJC can be determined by calculating the P′R interval. When the P′R interval is between 0.12 and 0.20 seconds, the beat is considered to be a PAC. When the P′R interval is calculated to be less than 0.12 seconds, the beat is a PJC. See Figure 4-2.

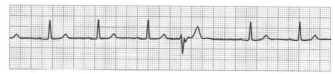

Figure 4-2   Normal sinus rhythm with premature junctional contraction.

Premature Junctional Contraction Interpretation Criteria

1. Rhythm: dependent on underlying rhythm, but irregular when PJC occurs
2. Rate: dependent on underlying rhythm's rate, usually 60–100 bpm
3. P′ waves: occur before, during, or after the QRS. Inverted when present in leads II, III, aVF
4. P′RI: when present, less than 0.12 sec
5. QRS I: less than 0.12 sec

Review Question

What criteria distinguish this rhythm from NSR?_____

[Inverted P wave before, during, or after QRS with beat occur-
ring once in a while. When P occurs before QRS, PRI less than
0.12 seconds. Irregular rhythm.]

Premature Junctional Contraction Care Measures

When identified as premature junctional contractions, the first step is to identify the effect of the rhythm on the patient's clinical signs and symptoms and establish the cause as being related to premature or escape causes. If the rhythm is asymptomatic with less than 10 bpm, no treatment is needed. When the rhythm is either symptomatic or occurring at a rate over 10 bpm, treatment of the cause is recommended to decrease irritability or promote automaticity of the higher pacemaker sites.

Premature Junctional Contraction Care Measures

- Assess impact of the rhythm on the patient's clinical signs and symptoms
- Prevent/treat the underlying cause
  - Educate the patient about lifestyle changes
    - Decrease caffeine intake
    - Smoking cessation
  - Refer to recreational drug rehabilitation programs
  - Assess serum digoxin levels. Adjust dosages for levels to be therapeutic between 0.9–1.5 ng/mL

— Assess electrolyte levels (potassium and magnesium). Adjust dosages for levels to be therapeutic

- Potassium: normal serum level 4.0–5.0 mEq/L, and 4.3–5.0 mEq/L in cardiac surgery patients
- Magnesium: normal serum level 1.8–2.4 mg/dL

— Treat the cardiac disease-related states

JUNCTIONAL ESCAPE RHYTHM (JER)

Junctional escape rhythm (JER) is a rhythm with sequential beats originating in the junctional tissue at the rate of 40 to 60 bpm. Each junctional beat flows simultaneously in two directions: (1) retrograde depolarization occurs as the impulse flows backward through the atria forming an inverted P′ wave with a shortened P′R interval, a missing P′ wave, or an inverted P′ wave after the QRS, which may change the appearance of the QRS; and (2) a normal or antegrade depolarization process through the ventricles eliciting a typical QRS complex and QRS interval of 0.06 to 0.12 seconds (Fig. 4-3).

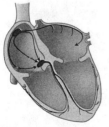 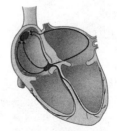

Normal Conduction
Pathway

Conduction Pathway in
Junctional Escape Rhythm

Figure 4-3   Conduction pathway in junctional escape rhythm.

Junctional Escape Rhythm Causes

The two main reasons for a junctional escape rhythm are with sinus bradycardia of less than 40 bpm or blockage of the impulse reaching the AV junctional tissue signaling the AV junction to initiate a rhythm. Blockage of the rhythm reaching the AV junctional tissue can occur with sinus block or sinoatrial arrest. In either scenario, the junctional tissue takes over as the pacemaker of the heart and initiates beats at its inherent rate of 40 to 60 bpm. Drugs and heart damage may lead to blockage of sinus and atrial impulses.

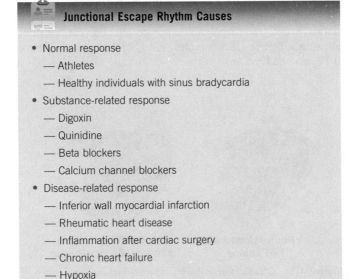

Junctional Escape Rhythm Causes

- Normal response
  — Athletes
  — Healthy individuals with sinus bradycardia
- Substance-related response
  — Digoxin
  — Quinidine
  — Beta blockers
  — Calcium channel blockers
- Disease-related response
  — Inferior wall myocardial infarction
  — Rheumatic heart disease
  — Inflammation after cardiac surgery
  — Chronic heart failure
  — Hypoxia

Junctional Escape Rhythm Assessment

Similar to sinus bradycardia, the junctional escape rhythm may be asymptomatic or may cause a decrease in cardiac output. REMEMBER: Cardiac output = heart rate × stroke volume; therefore as the heart rate slows down, the cardiac output may decrease. The risk for decreased cardiac output increases when the P′ is found during or after the QRS related to a loss of atrial kick, which prevents blood being ejected from the atria into the ventricles; therefore less blood moves out of the ventricles, with the ventricular contraction seen on the ECG by the QRS complex. The loss of atrial contraction immediately before the ventricular contraction accounts for a loss of approximately 30% of the blood usually ejected from the ventricles over a minute. A reduced cardiac output decreases the tissue perfusion and oxygen supplied to the heart, brain, and other organs in the body, leading to characteristic signs and symptoms of dizziness, dyspnea, chest pain, and/or hypotension.

Junctional Escape Rhythm Assessment

- Asymptomatic
- Dizziness
- Dyspnea
- Chest pain
- Hypotension

Junctional Escape Rhythm Interpretation Criteria

A junctional escape rhythm typically has a rate of 40 to 60 bpm with an inverted P′ wave found before, hidden within the QRS complex or after the QRS complex. An inverted P′ wave found before the QRS complex will have a P′R interval of less than

0.12 seconds. When the heart rate is slower than 40 bpm, the rhythm may be called junctional bradycardia. A heart rate of less than 40 bpm is considered to be bradycardic for junctional tissue, since the "normal" heart rate for junctional tissue is 40 to 60 bpm. See Figure 4-4.

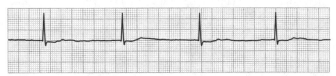

Figure 4-4 Junctional escape rhythm.

Junctional Escape Rhythm Interpretation Criteria

1. Rhythm: regular
2. Rate: 40–60 bpm
3. P' waves: occur before, during, or after the QRS. Inverted when present in leads II, III, aVF
4. P'RI: when present, less than 0.12 sec. If the P' wave falls in the QRS or after the QRS, the P'RI is not present.
5. QRS I: less than 0.12 sec

Review Question

What criteria distinguish this rhythm from NSR?_____

[Inverted P' wave before, during or after QRS. When P' before QRS, P'RI less than 0.12 seconds. Heart rate between 40–60 bpm.]

Junctional Escape Rhythm Care Measures

Once the rhythm is identified, the first step is to identify the effect of the rhythm on the patient's clinical signs and symptoms. If the rhythm is asymptomatic, determine and treat the cause such as adjusting digoxin dosages based on serum digoxin levels, discontinuing beta blockers and/or calcium channel blockers, and treating electrolyte imbalances. If the rhythm is symptomatic, follow the bradycardia algorithm suggested by the American Heart Association (see Appendix A).

Junctional Escape Rhythm Care Measures

- Assess impact of the rhythm on the patient's clinical signs and symptoms
- Treat symptomatic rhythm urgently
  - Oxygen
  - IV access
  - Atropine
  - Transcutaneous /transvenous pacing
  - Epinephrine or dopamine
- Prevent/treat the underlying cause
  - Assess serum digoxin levels. Adjust dosages for levels to be therapeutic between 0.9–1.5 ng/mL
  - Assess electrolyte levels (potassium and magnesium). Adjust dosages for levels to be therapeutic
    - Potassium: normal serum level 4.0–5.0 mEq/L, and 4.3–5.0 mEq/L in cardiac surgery patients
    - Magnesium: normal serum level 1.8–2.4 mg/dL
  - Discontinue beta blockers, calcium channel blockers or amiodarone
  - Treat the cardiac disease-related states

ACCELERATED JUNCTIONAL RHYTHM (AJR)

Accelerated junctional rhythm (AJR) is a rhythm with sequential beats originating in the junctional tissue at the rate of 60 to 100 bpm. Each junctional beat flows simultaneously in two directions: (1) retrograde depolarization occurs as the impulse flows backward through the atria forming an inverted P' wave with a shortened P'R interval, a missing P' wave, or an inverted P' wave after the QRS, which may change the appearance of the QRS; and (2) a normal or antegrade depolarization process through the ventricles eliciting a typical QRS complex and QRS interval of 0.06 to 0.12 seconds (Fig. 4-5).

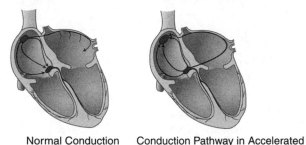

Normal Conduction   Conduction Pathway in Accelerated
Pathway   Junctional Rhythm

Figure 4-5   Conduction pathway in accelerated junctional rhythm.

Accelerated Junctional Rhythm Causes

The cause of accelerated junctional rhythm is due to irritability and enhanced automaticity of the junctional tissue. The irritability of the junctional tissue can be triggered by substances like digoxin, cardiac disease states, hypoxemia, or electrolyte disturbances. Although digoxin is known to decrease conductivity through the AV node, the drug also increases automaticity of cardiac tissue; especially in patients who are hypokalemic or hypomagnesemic. In cases of chronic obstructive pulmonary disease, a lack of oxygen to cells leads to sympathetic stimulation, which can cause the junctional tissue to increase its rate greater than the inherent rate of 40 to 60 bpm.

Accelerated Junctional Rhythm Causes

- Drug-related response
  — Digoxin
- Disease-related response
  — Inferior or posterior wall myocardial infarction
  — Rheumatic fever
  — Cardiac surgery
  — Chronic obstructive pulmonary disease (COPD)
  — Electrolyte disturbances
    - Hypokalemia
    - Hypomagnesemia

Accelerated Junctional Rhythm Assessment

Because the rate of this rhythm is within normal limits of 61 to 100 bpm, typically no clinical signs and symptoms are exhibited by the patient. Yet, in patients with P′ waves during or after the QRS, the loss of atrial kick can precipitate a decrease in cardiac output leading to milder signs and symptoms of fatigue, weakness, dizziness, and dyspnea.

Accelerated Junctional Rhythm Assessment

- Asymptomatic
- Fatigue
- Weakness
- Dizziness
- Dyspnea

Accelerated Junctional Rhythm Interpretation Criteria

An accelerated junctional rhythm typically has a rate of 61 to 100 bpm with an inverted P' wave found before, hidden within the QRS complex or after the QRS complex. An inverted P' wave found before the QRS complex will have a P'R interval of less than 0.12 seconds. See Figure 4-6.

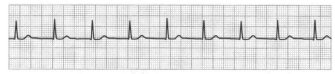

Figure 4-6   Accelerated junctional rhythm.

Accelerated Junctional Rhythm Interpretation Criteria

1. Rhythm: regular
2. Rate: 61–100 bpm
3. P' waves: occur before, during, or after the QRS. Inverted when present in leads II, III, aVF
4. P'RI: when present, less than 0.12 sec. If the P' wave falls in the QRS or after the QRS, the P'RI is not present
5. QRS I: less than 0.12 sec

Review Question

What criteria distinguish this rhythm from NSR?_____

[Inverted P' wave before, during, or after QRS. When P' before QRS, P'RI less than 0.12 seconds.]

Accelerated Junctional Rhythm Care Measures

After the rhythm has been interpreted, the next step is to identify the effect of the rhythm on the patient's clinical signs and symptoms. If the rhythm is asymptomatic, determine and treat the cause such as adjusting digoxin dosages based on serum digoxin levels, providing oxygen, and administering potassium chloride and magnesium replacements as needed based on serum levels. Two rules of thumb provide a guideline for potassium and magnesium replacements. For every 10 mEq/L of potassium given, expect a 0.1 mEq/L increase in the serum potassium level unless the patient is actively losing potassium from the body. The second rule of thumb is for every gram of magnesium sulfate administered, expect a 0.1 mg/dL rise in the serum magnesium level unless the patient is actively losing magnesium. Lastly, treat the disease states to decrease the irritability of the heart muscle.

Accelerated Junctional Rhythm Care Measures

- Assess impact of the rhythm on the patient's clinical signs and symptoms
- Prevent/treat the underlying cause
  — Assess serum digoxin levels. Adjust dosages for levels to be therapeutic between 0.9–1.5 ng/mL
  — Administer oxygen as needed based on SpO_2 levels. Keep SpO_2 >90%
  — Assess electrolyte levels (potassium and magnesium). Adjust dosages for levels to be therapeutic
    - Potassium: normal serum level 4.0–5.0 mEq/L, and 4.3–5.0 mEq/L in cardiac surgery patients
    - Magnesium: normal serum level 1.8–2.4 mg/dL
- Treat the cardiac disease-related states

JUNCTIONAL TACHYCARDIA (JT)

Junctional tachycardia (JT) is a rhythm with sequential beats origi-nating in the junctional tissue at the rate of 101 to 180 bpm. Each junctional beat flows simultaneously in two directions: (1) retrograde depolarization occurs as the impulse flows backward through the atria forming an inverted P′ wave with a shortened P′R interval, a missing P′ wave, or an inverted P′ wave after the QRS, which may change the appearance of the QRS; and (2) a normal or antegrade depolarization process through the ventricles eliciting a typical QRS complex and QRS interval of 0.06 to 0.12 seconds (Fig. 4-7).

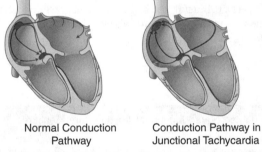

Normal Conduction   Conduction Pathway in
        Pathway   Junctional Tachycardia

Figure 4-7   Conduction pathway in junctional tachycardia.

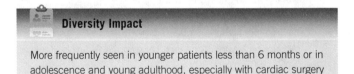

Diversity Impact

More frequently seen in younger patients less than 6 months or in adolescence and young adulthood, especially with cardiac surgery

Junctional Tachycardia Causes

The underlying issue with junctional tachycardia is irritability of the junctional tissue, which enhances the automaticity of the tis-sue so that the AV junction's pacemaker function overrides the

SA node pacemaker role. Again, digoxin is one of the main culprits initiating this rhythm, particularly if the patient is hypokalemic with potassium levels of less than 4.0 mEq/L. Inflammation from cardiac surgery or myocardial infarction may create irritable foci from the breakdown of cells and release of enzymes near the AV junction. Most typically, JT is seen when patients are being rewarmed after cardiac surgery when nodal inflammation and/or ischemia is present. Some types of congenital heart defects cause junctional ectopic tachycardia due to structural changes in the heart such as tetralogy of Fallot.

Junctional Tachycardia Causes

- Drug-related response
  - Digoxin
- Disease-related response
  - Inferior or posterior wall myocardial infarction
    Inflammation after cardiac surgery
  - Congenital heart defects in children
  - Electrolyte disturbances
    - Hypokalemia
    - Hypomagnesemia

Junctional Tachycardia Assessment

Similar to sinus tachycardia, junctional tachycardia may be asymptomatic or may cause a decrease in cardiac output. REMEMBER: Cardiac output = heart rate × stroke volume; therefore as the heart rate speeds up the cardiac output may decrease due to limited time for the ventricles to fill, which reduces the stroke volume.

More severe signs of decreased cardiac output typically exhibit themselves with this rhythm such as chest pain, hypotension, dyspnea, and confusion. Hemodynamic instability may occur related to a rapid pulse and low blood pressure. If the rhythm remains untreated, the patient may develop complications such as an extension of a myocardial infarction, chronic heart failure, and/or move into more dangerous ventricular dysrhythmias.

Junctional Tachycardia Assessment

- Asymptomatic—more rare
- Chest pain
- Dyspnea
- Hypotension
- Confusion

Junctional Tachycardia Interpretation Criteria

Junctional tachycardia has a rate of 101 to 180 bpm with an inverted P′ wave found before, hidden within the QRS complex or after the QRS complex. An inverted P′ wave found before the QRS complex will have a P′R interval of less than 0.12 seconds. Determination of the presence of a P′ wave may be difficult to distinguish when it falls after the QRS, particularly if the T wave obscures the P′ wave due to the rapid rate of this rhythm. See Figure 4-8.

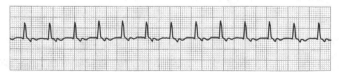

Figure 4-8   Junctional tachycardia.

Junctional Tachycardia Interpretation Criteria

1. Rhythm: regular
2. Rate: 101–180 bpm
3. P′ waves: occur before, during, or after the QRS. Inverted when present in leads II, III, aVF
4. P′RI: when present, less than 0.12 sec. If the P′ wave falls in the QRS or after the QRS, the P′RI is not present
5. QRS I: less than 0.12 sec

Review Question

What criteria distinguish this rhythm from NSR?_____

[Inverted P′ wave before, during, or after QRS.
When P′ before QRS, P′RI less than 0.12 seconds.
Heart rate 101–180 bpm.]

Junctional Tachycardia Care Measures

Digoxin toxicity is frequently the cause of this rhythm, especially if the patient is hypokalemic. If the patient is on digoxin, assess the serum digoxin and potassium levels. If the digoxin level is elevated, discontinue the drug and consider the need for administering a digoxin-binding drug as an antidote. Administration of beta blockers, calcium channel blockers, or amiodarone can help to control the heart rate and improve cardiac output, while considering how to treat the cause of the rhythm. In children, radiofrequency ablation is used when the junctional tachycardia is incessant with symptoms.

Junctional Tachycardia Care Measures

- Assess impact of the rhythm on the patient's clinical signs and symptoms
- Prevent/treat the underlying cause
  - Assess serum digoxin levels. Adjust dosages for levels to be therapeutic. Administer Digibind if serum digoxin level greater than 10 ng/mL
  - Assess electrolyte levels (potassium and magnesium). Adjust dosages for levels to be therapeutic
    - Potassium: normal serum level 4.0–5.0 mEq/L, and 4.3–5.0 mEq/L in cardiac surgery patients
    - Magnesium: normal serum level 1.8–2.4 mg/dL
- Reduce heart rate by administering beta blockers, calcium channel blockers, or amiodarone
- Radiofrequency ablation for children
- Treat the cardiac disease-related states

AV NODAL REENTRANT TACHYCARDIA (AVNRT)

AV nodal reentrant tachycardia (AVNRT) is usually preceded by a premature atrial contraction that initiates due to two conduction pathways through the AV node. Speed of impulse transmission and rate of recovery are different for each of the AV conduction pathways, leading to the formation of a loop with a rapid regular rhythm. The faster conduction pathway has a slower recovery period while the slower conduction pathway has a shorter recovery period. Onset and termination of the rhythm are sudden and have frequently been referred to as paroxysmal supraventricular tachycardia. P′ waves are usually not visible, as the impulse originates near the AV node spreading retrogradely through the atria and antegradely through the ventricles simultaneously. P'R interval is not present due to the absence of a P' wave. Conduction through the ventricles follows the bundle of His to the Purkinje fibers, resulting in a narrow QRS with an interval less than 0.12 seconds. Rhythm may last for seconds, hours, or days (Fig. 4-9).

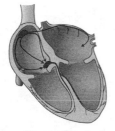 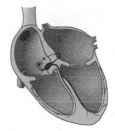

Normal Conduction   Conduction Pathway in AV Nodal
Pathway   Reentrant Tachycardia

Figure 4-9   Conduction pathway in AV nodal reentrant tachycardia.

Diversity Impact

More frequently seen in women than men, common in young adults (Olshansky et al., 2006).

AV Nodal Reentrant Tachycardia Causes

Most patients with this rhythm do not have structural damage to the heart. A familial tendency has been documented with an autosomal dominant trait (Hayes et al., 2004). Most precipitating factors of AVNRT are associated with lifestyle behaviors such as fear/anxiety/stress, sleep deprivation, caffeine, and hypoxia. Ninety percent of the AVNRT are seen after a premature atrial contraction with only 10% following a premature ventricular contraction; thus causes of these two extrasystolic beats may increase the risk of this rhythm. Both of these extrasystolic beats are frequently seen with sympathetic stimulation and are associated with mechanisms that cause irritability of the heart tissue.

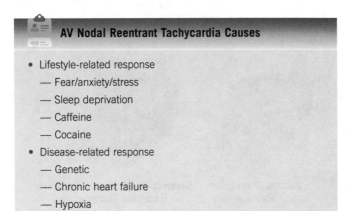

AV Nodal Reentrant Tachycardia Causes

- Lifestyle-related response
  — Fear/anxiety/stress
  — Sleep deprivation
  — Caffeine
  — Cocaine
- Disease-related response
  — Genetic
  — Chronic heart failure
  — Hypoxia

AV Nodal Reentrant Tachycardia Assessment

Because of the rapid heart rate, palpitations are commonly felt by patients. Syncope and hypotension could occur as the rhythm continues for longer periods of time, at faster rates, or upon onset of the rhythm due to the sudden decreased cardiac output. Chronic heart failure may occur due to the rapid heart rate and decreased amount of ventricular filling time leading to decreased ejection of blood from the heart. Chest pain and myocardial infarctions, particularly in patients with coronary artery disease or previous infarctions may occur due to the increased cardiac workload from the tachycardia.

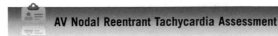

AV Nodal Reentrant Tachycardia Assessment

- Palpitations
- Syncope/hypotension

- Chest pain
- Chronic heart failure
- Myocardial infarction

AV Nodal Reentrant Tachycardia Interpretation Criteria

In an AVNRT, the rate is rapid between 150 to 250 bpm with the P′ wave hidden within the QRS complex or found immediately after the QRS complex. Since the electrical pathway through the ventricles follows the normal conduction pathway, the QRS complex is narrow with a QRS interval of 0.06 to 0.12 seconds (Figure 4-10).

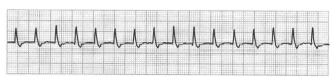

Figure 4-10   AV nodal reentrant tachycardia.

AV Nodal Reentrant Tachycardia Interpretation Criteria

1. Rhythm: usually regular
2. Rate: 150–250 bpm
3. P′ wave: hidden or inverted shortly after the QRS in leads II, III, aVF
4. P′RI: none
5. QRS I: usually less than 0.12 sec

AV Nodal Reentrant Tachycardia Care Measures

As is characteristic in treatment of dysrhythmias, the first step is to assess the effect of the rhythm on the patient's clinical signs and symptoms. Synchronized cardioversion is rarely necessary due to infrequency of this rhythm eliciting hemodynamic instability. The rhythm may be converted back to normal sinus rhythm through performance of vagal maneuvers such as carotid sinus massage (hospital use only), bearing down as if to have a bowel movement, or icy cold water facial immersion. Avoid the use of vagal maneuvers if the patient is hypotensive. If vagal maneuvers are ineffective in terminating the rhythm, then adenosine, beta blockers, and/or calcium channel blockers intravenously may be given to slow the heart rate. Following the American Heart Association Tachycardia with Pulses algorithm is recommended (see Appendix B). Radiofrequency catheter ablation is suggested for patients who refuse, are intolerant, or fail to respond to pharmacologic methods (Olshansky et al., 2006).

AV Nodal Reentrant Tachycardia Care Measures

- Assess impact of the rhythm on the patient's clinical signs and symptoms
- Determine stability of the patient
- Administer oxygen and obtain IV access

Stable

- Perform vagal maneuvers
- Administration of adenosine
- Administration of beta blockers and/or calcium channel blockers
- Prevent/treat the underlying cause
  — Educate the patient about lifestyle changes
    ▪ Counseling, stress reduction techniques, and anxiolytic agents

Unstable

- Perform synchronized cardioversion

- Sleep-inducing methods and hypnotics
- Decreasing caffeine intake
— Refer to recreational drug rehabilitation programs
• Radiofrequency catheter ablation

(2005 American Heart Association Guidelines for Cardiopulmonary Resuscitation and Emergency Cardiovascular Care, Part 2: Ethical Issues. *Circulation,* 2005;112(suppl IV):IV-6-IV-11.)

AV REENTRANT TACHYCARDIA (AVRT)

In AV reentrant tachycardia (AVRT), the impulse is transmitted via an accessory pathway that travels directly from the atria to the ventricles bypassing the AV node. A reentry circuit develops using various types of muscle fibers: Kent, Mahaim, and James. Each set of muscle fibers used translates to slightly different forms of AV reentrant tachycardia; for example, Kent fibers are involved in Wolff–Parkinson–White (WPW) syndrome. Advanced ECG interpretation by cardiologists can assist with the differentiation of the rhythms in the category of AV reentrant tachycardia. Here, the focus will be on the orthodromic reentrant tachycardia called Wolff–Parkinson–White syndrome. Orthodromic reentrant tachycardia is an electrical impulse which flows in the normal direction and accounts for 90% of AV reentrant tachycardias. Wolff–Parkinson–White syndrome is associated with an orthodromic reciprocating tachycardia, which occurs when the impulse travels from the atria through the AV node to the ventricles and then circles back to the atrium via an AV accessory pathway. Preexcitation of the ventricles occurs, meaning that the ventricles are stimulated earlier than expected if the normal conduction pathway was followed. From this conduction pathway evolves a narrow QRS with a tachycardia rate of 200 to 320 bpm. Frequently, AVRT is preceded by a premature atrial contraction or premature ventricular contraction. Due to the nature of WPW, atrial fibrillation is a serious risk factor that may lead to sudden cardiac death (Fig. 4-11).

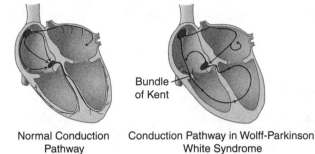

Normal Conduction   Conduction Pathway in Wolff-Parkinson
       Pathway   White Syndrome

Figure 4-11   Conduction pathway in Wolff–Parkinson–White
syndrome.

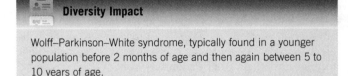

Diversity Impact

Wolff–Parkinson–White syndrome, typically found in a younger
population before 2 months of age and then again between 5 to
10 years of age.

AV Reentrant Tachycardia Causes

The root cause of AV reentrant tachycardia lies with the use of
accessory conduction pathways used during fetal development
and continuing to function after birth. Typically, after birth the
fetal conduction pathways stop functioning and the normal
conduction pathway assumes responsibility for conducting the
electrical impulses in the heart. When the fetal conduction
pathway or accessory pathways remain open and usable, three
different types of pre-excitation syndromes may develop based
on the location of the myocardial fibers and accessory pathways: Kent fibers, James bundle, and Mahaim fibers. Each of
these pathways are associated with various types of AV reentrant tachycardia.

AV Reentrant Tachycardia Causes

- Disease-related response
  — Congenital heart defects

AV Reentrant Tachycardia Assessment

Abrupt onset and termination of the rhythm and clinical signs and symptoms are similar to AV nodal reentrant tachycardia. The rhythm may disturb a patient's quality of life and the accessory pathway may lead to atrial fibrillation or atrial flutter, evolving into one of the more life-threatening supraventricular tachycardic rhythms.

AV Reentrant Tachycardia Assessment

- Palpitations
- Dyspnea
- Weakness
- Syncope/hypotension

AV Reentrant Tachycardia Interpretation Criteria

AV reentrant tachycardia is frequently concealed and not visible on an ECG. When visible, the rhythm is typically Wolff–Parkinson–White syndrome. Usually, WPW syndrome is not interpreted until the patient becomes tachycardic. When the patient is not tachycardic, the interpretation criteria for WPW are the presence of a delta wave, a short PR interval, and a QRS greater than 0.12 seconds. The preexcitation of the ventricles creates a slurring of the beginning of the R waves (delta wave) as the impulse stimulates the ventricles through the accessory pathway first rather than through the bundle of His and Purkinje fibers. A helpful method to determine the location site of the ECG disturbance is to give adenosine to slow the heart rate. If the patient "breaks" back to his or her previous cardiac rhythm, the cause of the supraventricular tachycardia is more likely a reentrant mechanism that involves the AV node, either AVNRT or AVRT. If the ventricular rate slows yet the atrial rate remains high, the rhythm is more likely atrial in origin. See Figure 4-12.

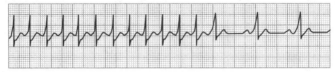

Figure 4-12   AV reentrant tachycardia.

AV Reentrant Tachycardia Interpretation Criteria

1. Rhythm: regular
2. Rate: 150–250 bpm
3. P′ waves: inverted P′ waves at end of QRS wave or early in ST segment
4. P′RI: none
5. QRS I: usually less than 0.12 sec

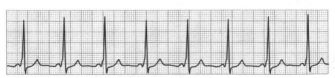

Figure 4-13   Wolff–Parkinson–White syndrome.

Wolff–Parkinson–White Syndrome Interpretation Criteria

1. Rhythm: regular
2. Rate: 60–100 bpm
3. P′ waves: upright, uniform, and round
4. PRI: less than 0.12 sec
5. QRS I: greater than 0.12 sec with delta wave present

AV Reentrant Tachycardia Care Measures

Comparable to other tachycardic rhythms in patients with a pulse, vagal maneuvers, adenosine, calcium channel blockers, and beta blockers are used for acute initial episodes. Following the American Heart Association Tachycardia with Pulses algorithm is recommended (see Appendix B). Wolff–Parkinson–White syndrome usually requires catheter ablation for treatment. In most patients, radiofrequency catheter ablation now eliminates the need for long-term drug therapy. While waiting for ablation, beta blockers, calcium channel blockers, procainamide, or amiodarone may be used to control the rate. Digoxin and verapamil may be contraindicated for some pathways of WPW syndrome related to an increased risk of sudden cardiac death. Consultation with a cardiologist is definitely recommended for this rhythm.

AV Reentrant Tachycardia Care Measures

- Assess impact of the rhythm on the patient's clinical signs and symptoms
- Determine stability of the patient
- Administer oxygen and obtain IV access

Stable	Unstable
• Perform vagal maneuvers	• Perform synchronized cardioversion
• Administration of adenosine	
• Administration of beta blockers, procainamide, and/or amiodarone	
• Radiofrequency catheter ablation	

(2005 American Heart Association Guidelines for Cardiopulmonary Resuscitation and Emergency Cardiovascular Care, Part 2: Ethical Issues. *Circulation,* 2005;112(suppl IV):IV-6-IV-11.)

PRACTICAL COMPARISON OF JUNCTIONAL RHYTHMS

Table 4-1 compares the junctional rhythms by rate which is the only feature which differentiates most of the junctional rhythms from each other.

Table 4-1   Comparison of Junctional Rhythms by Rate

Distin-guishing Features	NSR	PJC	JER	AJR	JT	AVNRT	AVRT
Rate (bpm)	60–100	Every once in a while	40–60	61–100	101–180	150–250	150–250

Tricks of the Trade

Once identified as junctional beats, comparison between the
junctional rhythms becomes easy as the main difference
between most of the junctional rhythms is the rate.

Table 4-2 on the next page compares the junctional rhythms to
each other and to NSR. Areas highlighted in red are features of
the rhythm which differentiates the rhythm from Normal Sinus
Rhythm.

Table 4-2   Practical Comparison of Junctional Rhythms

Distinguishing Features	NSR	PJC	JER
Rate (bpm)	60–100	Every once in a while	40–60
P′ wave	Upright uniform round	Inverted before, during, or after QRS	Inverted before, during, or after QRS
P′RI (sec)	0.12–0.20	< 0.12, when present	< 0.12, when present

NSR, normal sinus rhythm;
PJC, premature junctional contraction; JER, junctional escape rhythm; AJR, accelerated junctional rhythm; JT, junctional tachycardia; AVNRT, atrioventricular nodal reentrant tachycardia; AVRT, atrioventricular reentrant tachycardia.

AJR	JT	AVNRT	AVRT
61–100	101–180	150–250	150–250
Inverted before, during, or after QRS	Inverted before, during, or after QRS	Hidden or inverted after QRS	Hidden or inverted after QRS
< 0.12, when present	< 0.12, when present	None	None

REFERENCES

2005 American Heart Association Guidelines for Cardiopulmonary Resuscitation and Emergency Cardiovascular Care, Part 2: Ethical Issues. *Circulation*, 2005;112(suppl IV):IV-6 IV-11.

Hayes JJ, Sharma PO, Smith PN, et al. Familial atrioventricular nodal reentry tachycardia. *Pacing Clin Electrophysiol*. 2004; 27:73–76.

Olshansky B, Sandesara CM, Garg M, et al. Atrioventricular Nodal Reentrant Tachycardia (AVNRT): Differential diagnoses and workup. 2006. Available at: http://www.emedicine.com/med/topic2955.htm. Accessed October 7, 2008.

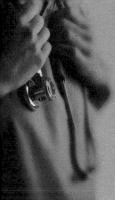

Chapter 5
VENTRICULAR RHYTHMS

Ventricular rhythms are initiated below the bundle of His in the ventricular tissue of the heart. Ventricular tissue has automaticity which may initiate beats at an inherent rate of 20 to 40 beats per minute (bpm). A few ventricular rhythms are tolerated well; yet many are life-threatening. Ventricular rhythms evolve when the higher pacemaker sites (SA node, atria, and AV junctional tissue) fail to function or are blocked; or with enhanced automaticity of the ventricular tissue. Each ventricular impulse flows through the ventricular tissue using an alternate pathway. The change in path way creates a wide, bizarre QRS with a prolonged QRS interval. With the change in pathway of ventricular depolarization, a change in ventricular repolarization also occurs, resulting in an opposite deflection of the T wave from the R wave.

PREMATURE VENTRICULAR CONTRACTIONS (PVCs)

Until interpreted, these ectopic beats are frequently and fondly referred to as "funny-looking beats." A premature ventricular contraction (PVC) is a beat that originates in the ventricular tissue either from irritability or as a "fail-safe" mechanism when the SA node, atria, and AV junctional tissue fail to initiate the beat or the beat is blocked in these higher pacemaker sites. If the PVC beat occurs before the expected time based on the patient's underlying rhythm with a short R-R interval between the preceding beat and the early PVC beat, the cause is attributable to irritability. When the PVC beat occurs later than the expected time based on the patient's underlying rhythm with a longer R-R interval between the preceding beat and the late PVC beat, the cause is attributable to a "fail-safe" mechanism due to a lack of performance by the SA node, atria, or AV junctional tissue. Fail-safe beats are occasionally referred to as ventricular escape beats. When a ventricular contraction is a solitary beat surrounded by other sinus beats, the differentiation between a premature beat and an escape beat becomes easy to view and important to understand when considering treatment. Despite the importance of the differentiation between prematurity and escape beats, in clinical practice solitary ventricular beats are referred to as PVCs. Each ventricular impulse flows through the ventricular tissue using an alternate pathway. The change in pathway creates a wide, bizarre QRS with a prolonged QRS interval. With the change in pathway of ventricular depolarization, a change in ventricular repolarization also occurs, resulting in an opposite deflection of the T wave from the R wave (Fig. 5-1).

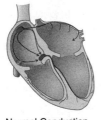 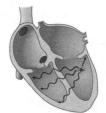

Normal Conduction Pathway   Conduction Pathway in Premature Ventricular Contraction

Figure 5-1   Conduction pathway in premature ventricular contractions.

Diversity Impact

May be seen in infants at birth, but are considered benign in children with normal structural hearts. Higher incidences of PVCs are found in men, African Americans, and the elderly.

Premature Ventricular Contraction Causes

PVCs may occur in healthy people without an identified cause. In athletes, the prevalence of frequent PVCs with structural and functional changes in the heart has been correlated with higher risks for fatal dysrhythmias. Typically, the causes of PVCs can be broken into two main categories: irritability and escape. Irritable causes of PVCs can be from increased sympathetic drive, electrolyte imbalances, acid–base imbalances, or structural damage to the cardiac tissue. Escape beats originate from failure or blockage of the SA node, atria, or AV junctional tissue to initiate a beat, leading to a pause that opens the opportunity for the ventricular tissue to become the pacer site of the heart. Causes of decreased automaticity of the higher pacer sites can be due to blockage from drugs such as beta blockers, calcium channel blockers, or digoxin; or may result from parasympathetic stimulation due to structural damage of the cardiac tissue from an inferior wall myocardial infarction/ischemia. Hypothermia slows the heart rate and provides an opportunity for the ventricles to initiate beats related to the previously mentioned fail-safe mechanism.

Premature Ventricular Contraction Causes

Irritability
- Normal response
  — Exercise
  — Fever
  — Hypovolemia
  — Fear/anxiety/stress
- Substance-related response
  — Lifestyle-related response

Escape
- Drug-related response
  — Beta blockers
  — Calcium channel blockers
  — Digoxin
- Disease-related response
  — Inferior wall myocardial infarction
  — Hypothermia

- ■ Caffeine
- ■ Alcohol
- ■ Nicotine
- ■ Methamphetamines/cocaine
  — Drug-related response
  - ■ Phenothiazines
  - ■ Tricyclic antidepressants
  - ■ Thrombolytics
- • Disease-related response
  — Electrolyte imbalances
  — Acid–base imbalances
  — Hypoxia
  — Acute coronary syndrome
  — Chronic heart failure

Premature Ventricular Contractions Assessment

Infrequent PVCs of less than ten per minute are considered to be clinically insignificant. An irregular pulse is generated related to the early or late response of the ventricular tissue to either irritability or lack of initiation of impulse by the higher pacemaker sites. The pulse may be weak or unable to be palpated due to an insufficient amount of ventricular filling time or an ineffective contraction due to initiation of the beat during the repolarization of the previous beat. Palpitations, a sensing of one's heart beating within the chest, may be felt, particularly with an increased frequency of PVCs per minute. As the number of PVCs per minute increases, the cardiac output may decrease, causing dizziness and hypotension. Some characteristics of PVCs affect the patient tolerance of the rhythm and affect the risk factor of conversion to a more dangerous dysrhythmia.

Premature Ventricular Contractions Assessment

- May be clinically insignificant
- Weak or absent pulse
  — Diminished heart sounds
  — Split S_2 heart sound
- Palpitations
- Decreased cardiac output
  — Dizziness
  — Hypotension

Premature Ventricular Contractions Interpretation Criteria

Because a PVC is a single beat, the underlying ECG rhythm must also be interpreted. An example of documentation of a rhythm might be: normal sinus rhythm with one premature ventricular contraction (NSR with a PVC). In premature ventricular contractions, the impulse originates in the ventricular tissue, and then the diffuse electrical activity spreads across both of the ventricles.

Premature ventricular contractions present with various characteristics. Because some characteristics are more dangerous than others, recognition and documentation of the characteristics are necessary to treat PVCs effectively. Characteristics can be broken into five components: configuration, pattern, frequency in a row, location, and R-on-T phenomenon.

PVCs that originate from the same ventricular site will look alike and are termed monomorphic or unifocal (Fig. 5-2). PVCs that originate from different sites in the ventricular tissue will appear different in shape and size on the ECG and are termed polymorphic or multifocal (Fig. 5-3). Polymorphic PVCs are considered more dangerous, as these ectopic beats reflect increased irritability of more areas of the ventricular tissue.

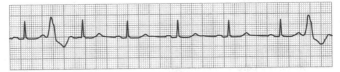

Figure 5-2   Normal sinus rhythm with monomorphic (unifocal) premature ventricular contractions.

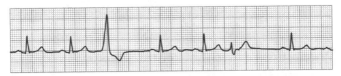

Figure 5-3   Normal sinus rhythm with polymorphic (multifocal) premature ventricular contractions.

The number of PVCs per minute can reflect the degree of irritability of the ventricular tissue. A greater number of PVCs typically reflects an increase in irritability of the ventricular tissue and a greater danger to the patient as the rhythm may progress to a potentially fatal rhythm of ventricular tachycardia. The frequency of PVCs may be documented in three separate ways: by a pattern of beatings, number in a row, and/or number per minute. Premature ventricular contractions may occur every other beat intermingled with the patient's underlying rhythm; this is termed bigeminy (Fig. 5-4). When PVCs occur after every third beat, this is termed trigeminy (Fig. 5-5) and after every fourth beat, quadrigeminy (Fig. 5-6). PVCs may also occur one right after another. Two sequential PVCs are called couplets (Fig. 5-7), three in a row are referred to as a salvo (Fig. 5-8), and four or more in a row are termed a run

(Fig. 5-9). Salvos and runs are also frequently referred to as short runs of ventricular tachycardia. As the number of PVCs per minute increases—such as with bigeminy, couplets, salvos, and runs—and when more than ten per minute are seen, the rhythm is considered to be more dangerous related to the potential for decreased cardiac output and the risk for conversion to ventricular tachycardia.

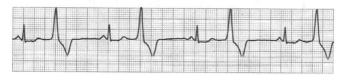

Figure 5-4   Normal sinus rhythm with bigminal premature ventricular contractions.

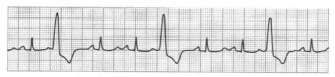

Figure 5-5   Normal sinus rhythm with trigeminal premature ventricular contractions.

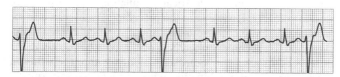

Figure 5-6   Normal sinus rhythm with quadrigeminal premature ventricular contractions.

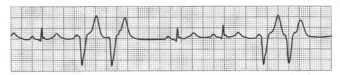

Figure 5-7   Normal sinus rhythm with couplets of premature ventricular contractions.

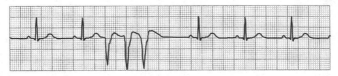

Figure 5-8   Normal sinus rhythm with salvo of premature ventricular contractions.

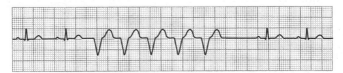

Figure 5-9   Normal sinus rhythm with run of premature ventricular contractions.

Another characteristic of PVCs can be the R-on-T phenomenon. An R-on-T phenomenon occurs when the PVC falls on the peak or downward slope of the T wave (Fig. 5-10). At this point, the ventricles may not be completely repolarized, and are therefore vulnerable to electrical stimulation. The response of striking the PVC R wave onto the preceding T wave can be conversion to a more dangerous rhythm of ventricular fibrillation. The R-on-T phenomenon tends to occur more frequently in the first 24 hours after a myocardial infarction without reperfusion treatments and in combination with an increased sympathetic drive. The ventricular tachycardia/fibrillation that may occur from the R-on-T phenomenon is usually not sustained.

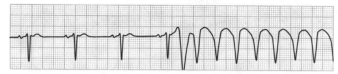

Figure 5-10 Normal sinus rhythm with R-on-T phenomenon in premature ventricular contractions leading to ventricular tachycardia.

Although more rarely described within clinical nursing practice, PVCs may be denoted as having a compensatory pause or being interpolated PVCs. A compensatory pause happens when the ventricles are unable to respond to the next P wave due to the refractory period from the PVC . A compensatory pause has occurred when the distance between three normal beats is the same as the distance between a sequence of a normal beat, PVC, and another normal beat (Fig. 5-11). An interpolated PVC is described as a PVC that sneaks in between two regularly scheduled sinus beats. Typically, the PR interval in the sinus beat following the interpolated PVC is longer than usual for that patient (Fig. 5-12).

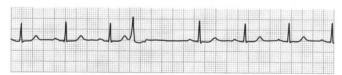

Figure 5-11 Normal sinus rhythm with compensatory pause in premature ventricular contraction.

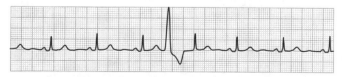

Figure 5-12 Normal sinus rhythm with interpolated premature ventricular contraction.

Premature Ventricular Contractions Interpretation Criteria

1. Rhythm: dependent on underlying rhythm, but may be irregular when PVC occurs
2. Rate: dependent on underlying rhythm's rate, usually 60–100 bpm
3. P waves: when present upright in ST segment or T wave, not associated with QRS
4. PRI: none
5. QRS I: wide, bizarre waveforms; greater than 0.12 sec. T wave in opposite direction of R wave

Characteristics of Premature Ventricular Contractions

- Configuration
  — Monomorphic (unifocal): PVCs similar in configuration
  — Polymorphic (multifocal): PVCs different in configuration
- Pattern
  — Bigeminal: PVCs every other beat
  — Trigeminal: PVCs every third beat
  — Quadrigeminal: PVCs every fourth beat
- Frequency in a row
  — Couplet: two PVCs in a row
  — Salvo: three PVCs in a row
  — Run: four or more PVCs in a row
- R-on-T phenomenon: PVC occurs on peak or downward slope of T wave
- Location
  — Compensatory: PVC found in space between two full sinus R-R intervals
  — Interpolated: PVC found between one sinus R-R interval

Danger Risks Associated with PVC Characteristics

- Polymorphic (multifocal)
- Couplets, salvos, runs
- Greater than 10 PVCs per minute
- R-on-T phenomenon
- Medically unstable patients

Review Question

What criteria distinguish this rhythm from NSR?_____

[Wide bizarre QRS with QRS interval greater than 0.12 seconds, beat occurs every once in a while]

Premature Ventricular Contractions Care Measures

When identified as premature ventricular contractions, the first step is to identify the effect of the rhythm on the patient's clinical signs and symptoms and establish the cause as being related to irritable or escape origins. If the rhythm is asymptomatic and does not meet the dangerous risk characteristics of PVCs, typically no treatment is needed. When the rhythm is symptomatic, the initial step is to treat the cause, such as providing counseling/medications for anxiety and stress, replacing electrolytes, correcting acid–base imbalances, administering oxygen for hypoxia, adjusting body temperature, and eliminating lifestyle and drug substances precipitating the rhythm. PVCs from myocardial ischemia and infarctions may be treated with beta blockers and/or amiodarone. Beta blockers slow the pulse by suppressing the SA node and prolonging the conduction through the AV node. Beta blockers are recommended for athletes, symptomatic PVCs, and recent myocardial infarctions. Amiodarone lengthens the action potential and refractory periods, which prolongs the PR and QT intervals, reducing the heart rate. Amiodarone is used when the PVCs are creating hemodynamic instability in the patient. Radiofrequency ablation sends electrical signals via a catheter to zap the irritable focus producing the PVCs. Ablative techniques are reserved only for patients with cardiomyopathy and a history of PVCs (Bogun et al., 2007).

Premature Ventricular Contractions Care Measures

- Assess impact of the rhythm on the patient's clinical signs and symptoms.
- Treat the cause.
- Asymptomatic, no treatment needed.
- Symptomatic
  — Oxygen
  — IV access
  — Beta blockers
  — Amiodarone
  — Radiofrequency ablation

IDIOVENTRICULAR RHYTHM (IVR)

A rhythm with sequential beats originating in the ventricular tissue at a rate of 20 to 40 bpm is an idioventricular rhythm (IVR). Each ventricular impulse flows through the ventricular tissue using an alternate pathway across both of the ventricles.

The change in pathway creates a wide, bizarre QRS with a prolonged QRS interval. With the change in pathway of ventricular depolarization, a change in ventricular repolarization also occurs, resulting in an opposite deflection of the T wave from the R wave. Idioventricular rhythm is also called the "dying" heart or an agonal rhythm due to its incidence in the last stages of advanced cardiac disease seen just prior to asystole (Fig. 5-13).

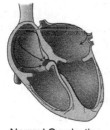   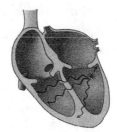

Normal Conduction
Pathway

Conduction Pathway in Idioventricular
Rhythm

Figure 5-13   Conduction pathway in idioventricular rhythm.

Idioventricular Rhythm Causes

The main reason for the cause of IVR is a failure to initiate or blockage of impulses from the SA node, atrial tissue, or AV junction. As a result, the automaticity of the ventricular tissue takes over as the main pacemaker of the heart. The beats are ventricular escape beats initiated as part of the protective mechanism of the heart. The inherent ventricular rate is 20 to 40 bpm. Drugs like digoxin, parasympathetic stimulation, and inferior wall myocardial damage can all prevent the higher pacer sites from functioning.

Idioventricular Rhythm Causes

- Drug-related response
  - Digoxin
- Disease-related response
  - Myocardial infarction
  - End-stage cardiac disease

Idioventricular Rhythm Assessment

The absence of an atrial kick from atrial contractions prior to ventricular contractions produces a significant decrease in cardiac output. The outcome of the reduction in adequate ejection of blood from the heart may yield symptoms of decreased tissue perfusion to many organs, leading to a decreased level of consciousness, skin mottling, and a backward blood flow, producing dyspnea and symptoms of heart failure. Usually after a period of time, the ventricles tire and the rhythm will deteriorate into a progressively more agonal rhythm, finally reaching asystole.

Idioventricular Rhythm Assessment

- Syncope/hypotension
- Dyspnea
- Mottling of skin
- Decreased level of consciousness

Idioventricular Rhythm Interpretation Criteria

In idioventricular rhythm, AV dissociation occurs meaning that the atria and the ventricles beat independently of each other.

As a result, P waves are either absent or totally unrelated to the QRS complex. Atrial rate and rhythm and the PR interval are unable to be determined due to inconsistent and independent atrial activity from ventricular activity. When P waves are present, the rhythm may be called third degree heart block. (See Chapter 6 for discussion of third degree heart block.) The ventricles initiate beats depicted by wide QRS complexes with QRS intervals greater than 0.12 seconds at a usually regular rate between 20 to 40 bpm. The T wave typically flows in the opposite direction from the R wave (Fig. 5-14).

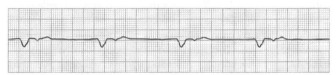

Figure 5-14   Idioventricular rhythm.

Idioventricular Rhythm Interpretation Criteria

1. Rhythm: usually regular
2. Rate: 20–40 bpm
3. P wave: may be present, but not associated with QRS
4. PRI: none
5. QRS I: wide, bizarre waveforms greater than 0.12 sec. T wave in opposite direction of R wave

Review Question

What criteria distinguish this rhythm from NSR?_____

[Wide bizarre QRS with QRSI greater than 0.12 seconds. Usually regular. Heart rate 20-40 bpm]

Idioventricular Rhythm Care Measures

As usual, the first step is to determine the impact of the rhythm on the patient's clinical signs and symptoms. When the rhythm is due to digoxin administration, discontinuing the drug or reducing the dose should treat the rhythm. If digoxin is not the cause of the rhythm, the next step is to evaluate the patient's level of consciousness. If the patient has mental capacity, the health care team should educate the patient and their family about the patient's health status and discuss the patient's wishes related to future health care. Two outcomes typically result from this discussion: either the decision is to maintain the patient in a full code status or to provide comfort care and prepare for the patient's death. If the decision is to continue all measures, atropine may be administered to increase the heart rate. Remember cardiac output = heart rate × stroke volume! A second action could be to pace transcutaneously. In addition, the patient may require intravenous fluids and vasopressors to maintain blood pressure. At no time should class IA antidysrhythmics (lidocaine and procainamide) be administered, as their action would be to suppress ventricular activity, leading to asystole. If the decision is to provide comfort care, follow the end-of-life protocol at your institution.

Idioventricular Rhythm Care Measures

- Assess impact of the rhythm on the patient's clinical signs and symptoms.
- Treat digoxin toxicity.
- Convene patient/family conference to discuss wishes related to advance directives.

Full Code
- Administer atropine.
- Attempt transcutaneous pacing.
- Administer fluid and vasopressors.

Comfort Care
- Provide comfort care measures.

ACCELERATED IDIOVENTRICULAR RHYTHM (AIVR)

Accelerated idioventricular rhythm (AIVR) initiates in the ventricular tissue with three or more ventricular beats in a row at a rate of 41 to 100 bpm, which is accelerated or faster than the inherent rate for ventricular beats. Each ventricular impulse flows through the ventricular tissue using an alternate pathway across both of the ventricles. The change in pathway creates a wide, bizarre QRS with a prolonged QRS interval. With the change in pathway of ventricular depolarization, a change in ventricular repolarization also occurs, resulting in an opposite deflection of the T wave from the R wave (Fig. 5-15).

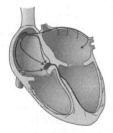 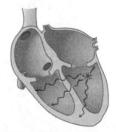

Normal Conduction Pathway

Conduction Pathway in Accelerated Idioventricular Rhythm

Figure 5-15   Conduction pathway in accelerated idioventricular rhythm.

Accelerated Idioventricular Rhythm Causes

Frequently, AIVR is seen immediately after a myocardial infarction or as a reperfusion dysrhythmia after thrombolytics or percutaneous coronary interventions. Another cause of AIVR may be drug related as an adverse effect from digoxin administration.

Accelerated Idioventricular Rhythm Causes

- Drug-related response
  — Successful thrombolytic therapy
  — Digoxin toxicity
- Disease-related response
  — Myocardial infarction
  — Electrolyte imbalances
  — Successful percutaneous coronary interventions

Accelerated Idioventricular Rhythm Assessment

The symptoms of decreased cardiac output correspond to the effects of the loss of an atrial kick. The absence of a P wave and its association to the QRS decreases ventricular filling and stroke volume, leading to the reduced amount of blood being forwardly ejected into the bloodstream. As a result, the classic symptoms of low cardiac output may be more readily observed, such as dizziness, dyspnea, chest pain, and hypotension.

Accelerated Idioventricular Rhythm Assessment

- Dizziness
- Dyspnea
- Chest pain
- Hypotension

Accelerated Idioventricular Rhythm Interpretation Criteria

In accelerated idioventricular rhythm, AV dissociation occurs meaning that the atria and the ventricles beat independently of each other. As a result, P waves are either absent or totally unrelated to the QRS complex. Atrial rate and rhythm and the PR interval are unable to be determined due to inconsistent and independent atrial activity from ventricular activity. When P waves are present, the rhythm may be called third degree heart block. (See Chapter 6 for discussion of third degree heart block.) The ventricles initiate beats depicted by wide QRS complexes with QRS intervals greater than 0.12 seconds at a usually regular rate between 41 to 100 bpm. The T wave typically flows in the opposite direction from the R wave. The main difference that distinguishes this rhythm from idioventricular rhythm or ventricular tachycardia is the ventricular rate (Fig. 5-16).

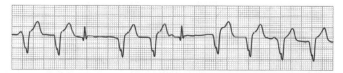

Figure 5-16   Accelerated idioventricular rhythm.

Accelerated Idioventricular Rhythm Interpretation Criteria

1. Rhythm: regular
2. Rate: 41–100 bpm
3. P wave: may be present, but not associated with QRS
4. PRI: none
5. QRS I: wide, bizarre waveforms greater than 0.12 sec. T wave in opposite direction of R wave

Review Question

What criteria distinguish this rhythm from NSR?_____

[*Wide, bizarre QRS! greater than 0.12 seconds.*
Usually regular. Heart rate 41–100 bpm]

Accelerated Idioventricular Rhythm
Care Measures

Typically, AIVR is a ventricular escape rhythm that evolves and disappears spontaneously with a rate higher than the patient's underlying sinus rhythm. Usually, treatment of AIVR is to observe and monitor the patient's hemodynamic stability. If the patient is digoxin toxic, the dose should be reduced or the drug discontinued. For serum digoxin levels greater than 10 ng/mL, especially in combination with hypokalemia, consider the need to administer Digibind, which is the antidote for digoxin toxicity. If symptomatic, atropine and/or transcutaneous pacing may be performed to incite the SA node to overrule the ventricular escape pacer site. Although rarely needed, an atrial pacer may be used for a hemodynamically unstable patient to stimulate the heart to support the pulse rate. Class IA antidysrhythmics again need to be withheld for two reasons: (1) AIVR is a protective rhythm and keeps the heart beating until the SA node or higher pacer site can again take over its responsibilities, and (2) AIVR is typically temporary and will resolve on its own.

Accelerated Idioventricular Rhythm Care Measures

- Assess impact of the rhythm on the patient's clinical signs and symptoms.
- Carefully and frequently observe the blood pressure, pulse, respirations and cardiac rhythm.

- Treat the cause.
- Symptomatic
  — Administer atropine 0.5–1 mg IV.
  — Attempt atrial pacing.

VENTRICULAR TACHYCARDIA (VT)

A rhythm of three or more sequential beats originating in the ventricles with a rate of greater than 100 per minute is ventricular tachycardia (VT). VT is a life-threatening rhythm initiated below the bundle of His in the ventricular tissue of the heart. Each ventricular impulse flows through the ventricular tissue using an alternate pathway. The change in pathway creates a wide, bizarre QRS with a prolonged QRS interval. The rhythm may be so rapid that T waves are not visible, and if visible, are deflected in the opposite direction of the R wave (Fig. 5-17).

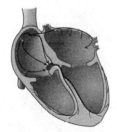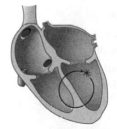

Normal Conduction
Pathway

Conduction Pathway in Ventricular
Tachycardia

Figure 5-17 Conduction pathway in ventricular tachycardia.

Diversity Impact

Rarely seen in children. May be seen with complex congenital heart defects and after heart surgery.

Ventricular Tachycardia Causes

Ventricular tachycardia most commonly arises from a reentry mechanism in myocardial ischemia and infarction. Electrolyte imbalances and acid–base imbalances may alter movement of cations across cell membranes, leading to increased irritability. Irritability of the ventricles may evolve from increased sympathetic stimulation due to lifestyle substances or drugs causing early or delayed afterdepolarizations. Torsades de pointes may evolve from end-stage heart disease, hypomagnesemia, or drugs that prolong the QT interval greater than 0.44 seconds (lidocaine, procainamide, amiodarone, antihistamines, antibiotics, antipsychotics).

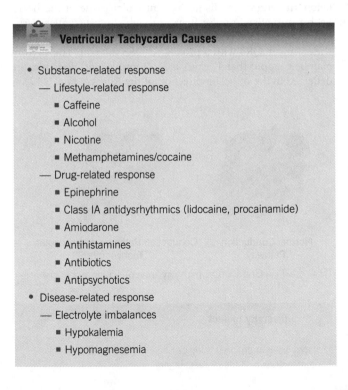

Ventricular Tachycardia Causes

- Substance-related response
  - Lifestyle-related response
    - Caffeine
    - Alcohol
    - Nicotine
    - Methamphetamines/cocaine
  - Drug-related response
    - Epinephrine
    - Class IA antidysrhythmics (lidocaine, procainamide)
    - Amiodarone
    - Antihistamines
    - Antibiotics
    - Antipsychotics
- Disease-related response
  - Electrolyte imbalances
    - Hypokalemia
    - Hypomagnesemia

— Acid–base imbalances
— Myocardial ischemia/infarction/coronary artery disease
— Chronic heart failure
— Trauma

Ventricular Tachycardia Assessment

No matter what, this rhythm is considered clinically significant and requires immediate treatment. Even when the rhythm is seen in an awake patient with a weak pulse, the potential for becoming unstable and deteriorating into cardiac arrest is extremely high. An atrial kick seen by a P wave preceding the QRS complex is absent in this rhythm. The loss of atrial kick and tachycardia results in severely decreased cardiac output leading to hypotension, pulselessness, and unresponsiveness. In rare patients, this rhythm is experienced chronically with minimal clinical effect.

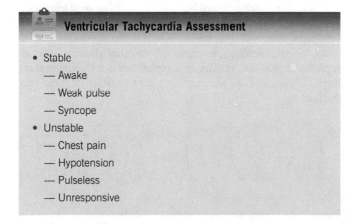

Ventricular Tachycardia Assessment

- Stable
  — Awake
  — Weak pulse
  — Syncope
- Unstable
  — Chest pain
  — Hypotension
  — Pulseless
  — Unresponsive

Ventricular Tachycardia Interpretation Criteria

Because some characteristics of ventricular tachycardia are more dangerous than others, recognition and documentation of the characteristics is necessary to treat ventricular tachycardia effectively. Characteristics can be broken into three components: shape, length of time in rhythm, and medical stability of the patient. Both monomorphic (Fig. 5-18) and polymorphic forms of ventricular tachycardia threaten the patient's life. In monomorphic VT, the ventricular beats are unifocal or arising from the same area of ventricular tissue and have a similar appearance for each QRS complex. In polymorphic ventricular tachycardia, the ventricular beats are multifocal or arise from different areas of ventricular tissue and have varying configurations of the QRS complex from beat to beat (Fig. 5-19). Occasionally, polymorphic ventricular tachycardia is seen in a particular pattern referred to as torsades de pointes. Often called "torsades," the rhythm is characterized by a "twisting of the point" or complexes that alternate every few beats between upward and downward deflections of the QRS. In nonsustained ventricular tachycardia, the rhythm is maintained for less than 30 seconds. When the rhythm continues for longer than 30 seconds in a sustained format, the reduced cardiac output decreases tissue perfusion to organs and places the patient in a life-threatening situation, leading quickly to medical instability and cardiac arrest. Differentiation of medical stability and instability by clinical signs and symptoms are seen in the previous table. At times, VT is difficult to distinguish from other rhythms such as supraventricular tachycardia in a patient with a bundle branch block. A 12-lead ECG may facilitate differentiation of these two rhythms.

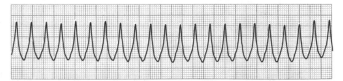

Figure 5-18   Monomorphic ventricular tachycardia.

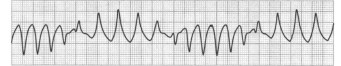

Figure 5-19   Polymorphic ventricular tachycardia, torsades de pointes.

Ventricular Tachycardia Interpretation Criteria

1. Rhythm: mostly regular for monomorphic. Regular or irregular for polymorphic
2. Rate: 101–250 bpm
3. P wave: not associated with QRS wave
4. PRI: none
5. QRS I: wide, bizarre waveforms greater than 0.12 sec

Characteristics of Ventricular Tachycardia

- Shape
  — Monomorphic: similar QRS waveform from beat to beat
  — Polymorphic: varying direction and amplitude of QRS waveform, altering every few beats, typically with higher rates between 200 and 250
- Length of time in rhythm
  — Nonsustained: lasting less than 30 sec, with spontaneous conversion to previous rhythm
  — Sustained: lasting longer than 30 sec
- Symptoms
  — Stable: awake, weak, palpitations
  — Unstable: hypotension and/or unresponsive, may be pulseless

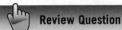
Review Question

What criteria distinguish this rhythm from NSR?_____

[Wide bizarre QRS with QRSI greater than 0.12 seconds. Usually regular. Heart rate 101–250 bpm]

Ventricular Tachycardia Care Measures

The first step is to assess the effect of the rhythm on the patient's clinical signs and symptoms. In the presence of a pulse with ventricular tachycardia, the administration of oxygen needs to be completed while simultaneously starting to consider the cause of the rhythm in the patient. Treatment of the cause of ventricular tachycardia will probably need to occur simultaneously with the administration of amiodarone 150 mg IV. Amiodarone acts by slowing the PR and QT intervals and the sinus node automaticity. Dosages of amiodarone may be given as needed until the maximum daily dose of 2.2 g/24 h is reached. Collaboration with a cardiologist is recommended with consideration of elective cardioversion if the VT continues. In the presence of torsades de pointes, magnesium sulfate 1 to 2 g is suggested to suppress the early after depolarizations by decreasing the movement of calcium into the cardiac cells (AHA, 2005). Following the Tachycardia with Pulses algorithm suggested by the American Heart Association is recommended when the patient has a pulse. See Appendix B.

In the absence of a pulse in ventricular tachycardia, basic life-support (BLS) protocol and oxygen administration needs to be initiated immediately. Pulseless ventricular tachycardia is a shockable rhythm; therefore the patient needs to be defibrillated with an automatic external defibrillator (AED) in the community or with a monophasic defibrillator at 360 J or a manual biphasic defibrillator at 200 J in the hospital or urgent care center. A pattern of defibrillation immediately followed by five cycles of cardiopulmonary resuscitation (CPR) continues until the code is called or the patient converts to a perfusing rhythm. As soon as intravenous or intraosseous access is obtained, 1 mg of epinephrine is given and may be repeated every 3 to 5 minutes as long as the rhythm continues. Epinephrine intensifies action at the alpha, beta$_1$, and beta$_2$ adrenergic receptor sites, causing vasoconstriction and bronchodilation (AHA, 2005). Vasopressin works as a non-adrenergic vasoconstrictor and is currently suggested by the American Heart Association algorithm guidelines; yet a study in the *New England Journal of Medicine* (Gueugniaud et al., 2008) finds no significant difference in patient outcomes between vasopressin and epinephrine versus epinephrine alone (see Evidenced-Based Practice). Other antidysrhythmics may also be used to attempt to convert the rhythm, such as amiodarone or lidocaine. Similar to VT with a pulse, magnesium may be used for torsades de pointes. As the pulseless arrest algorithm is being implemented, consideration and treatment of possible causes of the rhythm should be put into action (AHA, 2005). Following the Pulseless Arrest algorithm suggested by the American Heart Association is recommended when the patient is pulseless (see Appendix C). For patients who frequently experience ventricular tachycardia or who have arrested, an automatic cardioverter-defibrillator may be recommended.

Clinical Alert

Artifact from patient movement may represent itself on an ECG as ventricular tachycardia. Avoid misdiagnosis by palpating the pulse before using manual defibrillator.

Evidenced-Based Practice

The combination of catecholamines (epinephrine) and vaso-pressin seemed logical to improve perfusion and decrease adverse effects in cardiopulmonary arrests; yet positive results of previous studies were based on animals and small subgroups of humans. A multicenter clinical trial was created to investigate the effects of vasopressin and epinephrine versus epinephrine alone in patients found in the field with ventricular fibrillation, pulseless electrical activity, and asystole related to the patient's ability to survive to hospital admission, achieve spontaneous circulation, survive to hospital discharge, achieve good neurologic recovery, and survive to a 1-year end-point. A sample of 2,894 adults were randomly assigned into the experimental and control groups using a double-blind research method, with 1,442 in the vasopressin and epinephrine group and 1,452 in the epinephrine alone group. Although no statistically significant difference was found between the two groups, epinephrine alone appeared to have slightly better outcomes than the combination of vasopressin and epinephrine. Epinephrine remains the only drug in cardiopulmonary arrests that is supported with evidenced-based practice.

Outcomes	Epinephrine and Vasopressin (%)	Epinephrine Alone(%)
Survival to hospital admission	20.7	21.3
Return of spontaneous circulation	28.6	29.5
Survival to hospital discharge	1.7	2.3
Good neurologic recovery	37.5	51.5
Survival to 1 year	1.3	2.1

(Gueugniaud et al., 2008)

Ventricular Tachycardia Care Measures

- Assess impact of the rhythm on the patient's clinical signs and symptoms.
- Determine presence/absence of pulse.

Pulse Present

- Administer oxygen.
- Treat reversible causes.
- For regular rhythm, administer amiodarone 150 mg IV over 10 min. May repeat as needed to maximum dose of 2.2 g/24 h, and prepare for synchronized cardioversion,
- For irregular rhythm believed to be polymorphic VT, collaborate with cardiologist and consider magnesium sulfate 1–2 g for torsades de pointes.

Pulse Absent

- Follow basic life-support algorithm.
- Administer oxygen.
- Determine if a shockable rhythm.
- If VT, shock with 360 J using monophasic defibrillator or 200 J using manual biphasic defibrillator.
- Immediately restart CPR—do 5 cycles.
- Reassess rhythm. If shockable, repeat defibrillation.
- Immediately restart CPR—do 5 cycles.
- Before or after second defibrillation, administer epinephrine 1 mg IV/IO as soon as access available. May repeat every 3–5 min.
- Reassess rhythm. If shockable, repeat defibrillation and continue above process
- Consider amiodarone 300 mg IV/IO followed by repeat of 150 mg IV/IO or lidocaine loading doses of 1–1.5 mg/kg followed by 0.5–0.75 mg/kg up to 3 mg/kg.
- Consider administering magnesium for torsades de pointes.
- Treat reversible causes.

(2005 American Heart Association Guidelines for Cardiopulmonary Resuscitation and Emergency Cardiovascular Care, Part 2: Ethical Issues. *Circulation*, 2005;112(suppl IV):IV-6-IV-11.)

VENTRICULAR FIBRILLATION (VF)

Ventricular fibrillation (VF) is a rhythm initiated in the ventricles with a totally chaotic baseline without a distinguishable P, QRS, or T wave. Rapid firing of impulses simultaneously within the ventricles results in a lack of time for depolarization and repolarization to occur, producing a quivering of the ventricles, no ventricular contraction, and no cardiac output. Within seconds, the patient starts to die due to a complete lack of circulatory blood flow to organs. If untreated, the patient will die. Ventricular fibrillation is the main cause of sudden cardiac death (Fig. 5-20).

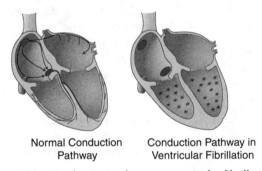

Normal Conduction   Conduction Pathway in
Pathway   Ventricular Fibrillation

Figure 5-20   Conduction pathway in ventricular fibrillation.

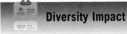

Diversity Impact

Ethnic differences may account for lower survival rates of black and Hispanic patients due to the underlying cause of the ventricular fibrillation (Galea et al., 2007). A higher incidence of sudden cardiac death is seen in men and the elderly.

Ventricular Fibrillation Causes

The causes of ventricular fibrillation arise from increased automaticity of the ventricular tissue or a reentry mechanism that is incomplete. As is expected, the most common cause is coronary artery disease, which may be associated with a myocardial infarction. Acid–base and electrolyte imbalances lead to irritability from movement of anions across the cardiac cell membranes during depolarization and repolarization.

Ventricular Fibrillation Causes

- Disease-related response
  - Myocardial ischemia/infarction/coronary artery disease
  - Acid–base imbalance
  - Electrolyte imbalance
    - Hypokalemia
    - Hyperkalemia
    - Hypercalcemia
    - Hypomagnesemia
  - Hypothermia
  - Electric shock

Ventricular Fibrillation Assessment

A patient in ventricular fibrillation will exhibit pulselessness, agonal to apneic breathing, and be unresponsive due to the lack of ventricular contractions, absence of forward movement of blood, and resulting decrease in tissue perfusion to organs. Similarly to pulseless ventricular tachycardia, a cardiac arrest has occurred when the patient exhibits this rhythm.

Ventricular Fibrillation Assessment

- Pulselessness
- Agonal to apneic breathing
- Unresponsive

Clinical Alert
Shivering, loose leads, and interference from electrical equipment may mimic ventricular fibrillation. Verify VF and assess impact of rhythm on patient's clinical signs and symptoms before intervening.

Ventricular Fibrillation Interpretation Criteria

The chaotic baseline may appear as coarse or fine waves. Coarse waves are more irregular and have a higher amplitude than fine waves. Coarse waves may disintegrate into fine fibrillatory waves prior to asystole. See Figure 5-21 for coarse VF and Figure 5-22 for fine VF.

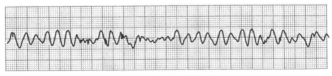

Figure 5-21   Coarse ventricular fibrillation.

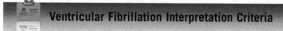

Figure 5-22   Fine ventricular fibrillation.

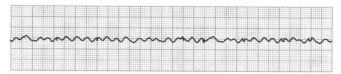

Ventricular Fibrillation Interpretation Criteria

1. Rhythm: Fine to coarse chaotic baseline
2. Rate: Unable to determine
3. P wave: None
4. PRI: None
5. QRS I: None

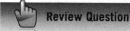

Review Question

What criterion distinguishes this rhythm from NSR?_____

[Totally chaotic baseline]

Ventricular Fibrillation Care Measures

Basic life-support protocol and oxygen administration need to be initiated immediately. Ventricular fibrillation is a shockable rhythm; therefore the patient needs to be defibrillated with an AED in the community or with a monophasic defibrillator at 360 J or a manual biphasic defibrillator at 200 J in the hospital or urgent care center. A pattern of defibrillation immediately followed by five cycles of CPR continues until the code is called or the patient converts to a perfusing rhythm 2005 (AHA, 2005). Coarse fibrillatory waves are more receptive to defibrillation than fine waves. The main focus of care for ventricular fibrillation is defibrillation and CPR. The goal of defibrillation is to depolarize the cardiac muscle at one moment in time to interfere with reentrant dysrhythmias and create an opportunity for the SA node, atrial tissue, or junctional tissue to again become the pacemaker of the heart. Guidelines for treatment of cardiac arrest may change for the performance of CPR in the field in the future (see Evidenced-Based Practice). Once intravenous or intraosseous access is established, medications can be administered following the pulseless arrest algorithm—epinephrine, vasopressin, amiodarone, lidocaine (EVAL). Amiodarone is considered superior to lidocaine, yet lidocaine is used when amiodarone is unavailable (Dorian et al., 2002). Similar to VT with a pulse, magnesium, 1 to 2 grams may be used for torsades de pointes. As the pulseless arrest algorithm is being implemented, the consideration and treatment of possible causes of the rhythm should be put into action.   Following the Pulseless Arrest algorithm suggested by the American Heart Association is recommended (see Appendix C). For recurrent ventricular fibrillation, amiodarone initial boluses are followed by a continuous IV drip of 1 mg/min for 6 hours and then 0.5 mg/min for 18 hours. The patient in ventricular fibrillation will die in 8 to 10 minutes if treatment has not been initiated.

Ventricular Fibrillation Care Measures

- Follow basic life-support algorithm.
- Administer oxygen.
- Determine if a shockable rhythm.
- If VF, shock with 360 J using monophasic defibrillator or 200 J using manual biphasic defibrillator.

- Immediately restart CPR—do 5 cycles.
- Reassess rhythm. If shockable, repeat defibrillation.
- Immediately restart CPR—do 5 cycles.
- Before or after second defibrillation, administer epinephrine 1 mg IV/IO as soon as access available. May repeat every 3–5 min.
- Reassess rhythm. If shockable, repeat defibrillation and continue above process.
- Consider amiodarone 300 mg IV/IO followed by repeat of 150 mg IV/IO or lidocaine loading dose of 1–1.5 mg/kg followed by 0.5–0.75 mg/kg up to 3 mg/kg.
- Consider administering magnesium for torsades de pointes.
- Treat reversible causes.

(2005 American Heart Association Guidelines for Cardiopulmonary Resuscitation and Emergency Cardiovascular Care, Part 2: Ethical Issues. *Circulation,* 2005;112(suppl IV):IV-6-IV-11.)

Evidenced-Based Practice

In this scientific advisory, several barriers to CPR performance of witnessed cardiac arrests are identified as limiting factors affecting survival rates: fears of disease transmission, fear of harming the victim, and unwillingness to perform mouth-to-mouth resuscitation. It is believed that the benefit of initial elimination of mouth-to-mouth resuscitation from CPR guidelines for witnessed adult cardiac arrest could increase the likelihood of bystander action and performance of CPR and outweigh the risks. The technique of "hands-only" CPR was developed for use by untrained or unconfident bystanders in witnessed arrests until EMT or AED arrives at scene.

(Sayre et al., 2008)

PULSELESS ELECTRICAL ACTIVITY (PEA)

Pulseless electrical activity (PEA) is a rhythm that presents with the ECG pattern visible in many other rhythms, but without a pulse. A frequent reminder in educational programs is to remember to look at the patient's signs and symptoms, not just the data from laboratory or diagnostic tests such as an ECG. A critical step in this situation! Because the patient looks on the monitor or 12-lead ECG as if there is no immediate need for intervention, the situation is misleading unless a patient assessment is completed. The electrical activity of the heart is present, but the mechanical ability of the heart to contract is unable to function. This situation is considered a cardiac arrest and requires immediate intervention to prevent death (Fig. 5-23). This rhythm was previously known as electromechanical dissociation (EMD).

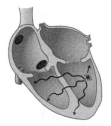
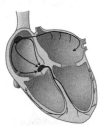

Possibly
Conduction Pathway of Idioventricular Rhythm, but without a Pulse

Possibly
Normal Conduction Pathway but without a Pulse

Figure 5-23   Conduction pathway in pulseless electrical activity.

Diversity Impact

Unknown reason, but more commonly seen in women than men. Higher incidence with a poorer prognosis found in the elderly.

Pulseless Electrical Activity Causes

Severe cardiac disease can result in an inability of the heart muscle to respond with contraction to the electrical stimulus. Several causes of PEA are reversible when treated in a timely manner. Hypovolemia and hypoxia are two of the main reversible causes of PEA. For example, a narrow complex tachycardia frequently is seen with dehydration. In severe cases of volume depletion, the decreased intravascular volume may be so drastic that a pulseless state evolves, resulting in PEA. Other contributing factors to the development of pulseless electrical activity have been categorized by the American Heart Association as the 6 Hs and 5 Ts to promote memory and use in practice.

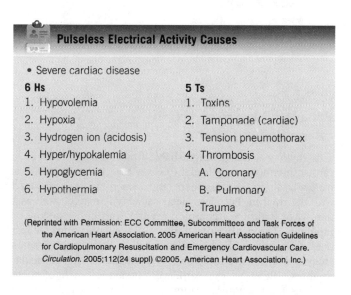

Pulseless Electrical Activity Causes

- Severe cardiac disease

6 Hs	5 Ts
1. Hypovolemia	1. Toxins
2. Hypoxia	2. Tamponade (cardiac)
3. Hydrogen ion (acidosis)	3. Tension pneumothorax
4. Hyper/hypokalemia	4. Thrombosis
5. Hypoglycemia	A. Coronary
6. Hypothermia	B. Pulmonary
	5. Trauma

(Reprinted with Permission: ECC Committee, Subcommittees and Task Forces of the American Heart Association. 2005 American Heart Association Guidelines for Cardiopulmonary Resuscitation and Emergency Cardiovascular Care. *Circulation.* 2005;112(24 suppl) ©2005, American Heart Association, Inc.)

Pulseless Electrical Activity Assessment

Although electrical activity is present when PEA is present, no functional activity exists, resulting in total cessation of the circulatory blood flow, no cardiac output, and no tissue perfusion to organs. A Doppler ultrasound is recommended to determine the absence of pulse versus a pulse which is difficult to palpate. Death will occur in 8 to 10 minutes without intervention.

Pulseless Electrical Activity Assessment

- Pulselessness
- No blood pressure
- Apnea
- Comatose

Pulseless Electrical Activity Interpretation Criteria

This rhythm is not distinguishable from other rhythms on a cardiac monitor or 12-lead ECG, yet the circumstances dramatically alter the assessment and care measures associated with the rhythm. Pulseless electrical activity may be seen as a narrow or wide QRS complex rhythm with either a slow or rapid rate. The rhythm that appears on the monitor may reflect one of the many rhythms already discussed, such as sinus tachycardia, supraventricular tachycardia, and idioventricular rhythms. (Refer to the earlier discussion of each of these rhythms for the interpretation criteria.) With each of these rhythms, no pulse is able to be palpated even though a pulse would be expected based on the rhythm seen on the monitor. The key to interpreting this rhythm is the absence of a pulse! See Figure 5-24.

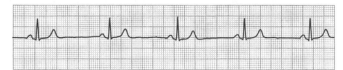

Figure 5-24   Pulseless electrical activity (rhythm without a pulse).

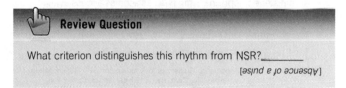

Review Question

What criterion distinguishes this rhythm from NSR?_____

[Absence of a pulse]

Pulseless Electrical Activity Care Measures

Even though the rhythm on the cardiac monitor appears to be commensurate with life, the first step is to identify the effect of the rhythm on the patient's clinical signs and symptoms. In the case of PEA, no pulse will be palpated, making this a critical life-threatening situation! Basic life support and oxygen need to be administered immediately. When either IV or IO access is available, epinephrine may be administered at 1 mg every 3 to 5 minutes to intensify action at the alpha, beta$_1$, and beta$_2$ adrenergic receptor sites causing vasoconstriction and bronchodilation. Atropine may be given at 1 mg every 3 to 5 minutes up to a total of 3 mg for the patient with a bradycardic rhythm. Once these measures have been started, the main course of action is to assess and treat for reversible causes (AHA, 2005). Since the two main culprits leading to this situation are hypovolemia and hypoxia, the administration of normal saline or lactated ringers IV boluses and determination of adequate oxygenation are typically critical in caring for this patient. Other sources of PEA that need to be considered and rapidly treated are the Hs and Ts listed earlier under "Pulseless Electrical Activity Causes." See Appendix C.

Pulseless Electrical Activity Care Measures

- Follow basic life-support algorithm.
- Administer oxygen.
- If pulseless electrical activity, DON'T shock!
- Perform 5 cycles of CPR repeatedly following the BLS algorithm.
- Administer epinephrine 1 mg IV/IO as soon as access available. May repeat every 3–5 min.
- May also administer atropine 1 mg IV/IO every 3–5 min up to 3 mg.
- Treat reversible causes. Review 6 Hs and 5 Ts.

(2005 American Heart Association Guidelines for Cardiopulmonary Resuscitation and Emergency Cardiovascular Care, Part 2: Ethical Issues. *Circulation*, 2005;112(suppl IV):IV-6-IV-11.)

ASYSTOLE

Characteristically, asystole is known as "flat line." On the ECG, the stylus portrays a flat line, indicating no electrical activity in the heart, which indicates a lack of cardiac output and no pulse. Within seconds, the patient starts to die due to a complete lack of circulatory blood flow to organs. If untreated, the patient will die (Fig. 5-25).

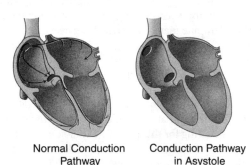

Normal Conduction   Conduction Pathway
Pathway   in Asystole

Figure 5-25   Conduction pathway in asystole.

Diversity Impact

More frequently seen in women than men, and in children than adults, as a presenting form of cardiac arrest (Caggiano, 2008).

Asystole Causes

The rhythm may be seen briefly after synchronized cardioversion, defibrillation, or the administration of medications in treatment of tachycardia. With each of these treatments, the premise behind the intervention is to completely stop the heart from beating and assume that the SA node will resume its function. Other causes of asystole are similar to PEA including the 6 Hs and 5 Ts.

Asystole Causes

- Therapy-related response
  — Synchronized cardioversion
  — Defibrillation
  — Drugs to convert tachycardia
- Disease-related response

6 Hs	**5 Ts**
1. Hypovolemia	1. Toxins
2. Hypoxia	2. Tamponade (cardiac)
3. Hydrogen ion (acidosis)	3. Tension pneumothorax
4. Hyper/hypokalemia	4. Thrombosis
5. Hypoglycemia	A. Coronary
6. Hypothermia	B. Pulmonary
	5. Trauma

(Reprinted with Permission: ECC Committee, Subcommittees and Task Forces of the American Heart Association. 2005 American Heart Association Guidelines for Cardiopulmonary Resuscitation and Emergency Cardiovascular Care. *Circulation.* 2005;112(24 suppl) ©2005, American Heart Association, Inc.)

Asystole Assessment

The first step is to assess the impact of the rhythm on the clinical signs and symptoms. If the patient has a pulse, the rhythm is NOT asystole. Pulselessness, apnea, and a comatose state evolve within seconds of onset of this rhythm due to a lack of circulating blood flow to the vital organs.

Asystole Assessment

- Pulselessness
- Apnea
- Comatose

Clinical Alert
Disconnection from the cardiac monitor or ECG leads may appear to be asystole. Assess lead electrodes, connections, and impact of rhythm on patient's clinical signs and symptoms before intervening.

Asystole Interpretation Criteria

All pacemaker sites in the heart have either failed to generate a beat or have been blocked from conducting the beat. Although typically not present, P waves may be seen without a ventricular response; referred to as ventricular standstill. Asystole is represented by a flat line on the monitor. Be careful that electrodes or leads have not been disconnected. It is recommended to check the rhythm in two different leads to verify the existence of asystole versus lead malfunction or fine ventricular fibrillation. See Figure 5-26.

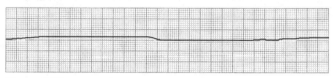

Figure 5-26 Asystole.

Asystole Interpretation Criteria

1. Rhythm: none
2. Rate: none
3. P wave: typically, not present
4. PRI: none
5. QRS I: none

Review Question

What criterion distinguishes this rhythm from NSR?_____

[flat line]

Asystole Care Measures

Immediate treatment may revive the patient from this cardiac death state. The algorithm recommended by the American Heart Association is the same one as that used for pulseless electrical activity. Similar to PEA, recognition and treatment of the reversible causes of asystole is critical once advanced cardiac life-support measures have been initiated. Atropine is no longer recommended for the treatment of asystole in infants and children, but is still used with adults. Following the Pulseless Arrest algorithm suggested by the American Heart Association is recommended (see Appendix C).

Asystole Care Measures

* Follow basic life-support algorithm.
* Administer oxygen.
* If asystole, DON'T shock!
* Perform 5 cycles of CPR repeatedly following the BLS protocol.
* Administer epinephrine 1 mg IV/IO as soon as access available. May repeat every 3–5 min.
* May also administer atropine 1 mg IV/IO every 3–5 min up to 3 mg.
* Treat reversible causes. Review 6 Hs and 5 Ts.

(2005 American Heart Association Guidelines for Cardiopulmonary Resuscitation and Emergency Cardiovascular Care, Part 2: Ethical Issues. *Circulation*, 2005;112(suppl IV):IV-6-IV-11.)

PRACTICAL COMPARISON OF VENTRICULAR RHYTHMS

Table 5-1 compares the ventricular rhythms to each other and to NSR. Areas highlighted in red are features of the rhythm which differentiates the rhythm from Normal Sinus Rhythm.

Table 5-1 Practical Comparison of Ventricular Rhythms

Distinguishing Features	NSR	PVC	IVR	AIVR	VT	VF	Asystole
Rhythm	Regular	Irregular when beat occurs	Usually regular	Regular	Usually regular	Chaotic baseline	None
Rate	60-100	Usually 60-100	20-40	41-100	101-250	Unable to determine	None
P waves	Upright Uniform Round	If present, not related to QRS	If present, not related to QRS	If present, not related to QRS	Not related to QRS	None	None
PRI	0.12-0.20	None	None	None	None	None	None
QRS l	<0.12	Wide, bizarre, >0.12	Wide, bizarre, >0.12	Wide, bizarre, >0.12	Wide, bizarre, >0.12	None	None
Pulse	Strong	Weak with beat	Weak	Weak	Weak or None	None	None

PEA may vary dependent on electrical rhythm; yet distinguishing feature is pulse unable to be palpated.

REFERENCES

2005 American Heart Association Guidelines for Cardiopulmonary Resuscitation and Emergency Cardiovascular Care, Part 2: Ethical Issues. *Circulation,* 2005;112(suppl IV):IV-6-IV-11.

Bogun F, Crawford T, Reich S, et al. Radiofrequency ablation of frequent, idiopathic premature ventricular complexes: comparison with a control group without intervention. *Heart Rhythm.* 2007;4:863–867.

Caggiano R. Asystole. Retrieved on September 24, 2008 from http://www.emedicine.com/EMERG/topic44.htm.

Dorian P, Cass D, Schwartz B, Cooper R, Gelaznikas R, Barr A. Amiodarone as compared with lidocaine for shock-resistant ventricular fibrillation. *N Engl J Med.* 2002;346:884–890.

Galea S, Blaney S, Nandi A, et al. Explaining racial disparities in incidence of and survival from out-of-hospital cardiac arrest. *Am J Epidemiol.* 2007;166 (5):534–543. Retrieved on September 24, 2008 from http://aje.oxfordjournals.org/cgi/content/full/kwm102v1.

Gueugniaud P, David J, Chanzy E, et al. Vasopressin and epinephrine versus epinephrine alone in cardiopulmonary resusucitation. *N Engl J Med.* 2008;359:21–30.

Sayre MR, Care DM, Potts J. Hands-only (compression-only) cardiopulmonary resuscitation: A call to action for bystander response to adults who experience out-of-hospital sudden cardiac arrest. *Circulation.* 2008;117:2162–2167.

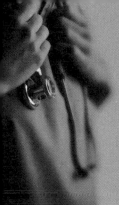

Chapter 6
ATRIOVENTRICULAR HEART BLOCKS

Atrioventricular (AV) heart blocks are rhythms caused by delays, incomplete or complete blocks of the electrical impulse at the AV node. The rhythm originates at the SA node and follows the normal electrical conduction pathway through the atria to the AV node. At the AV node, the impulse is either slowed in its conduction, incompletely blocked, or completely blocked from being conducted through the AV node. If the impulse is delayed, normal conduction through the ventricles displayed by a narrow QRS I will eventually be observed. If the impulse is incompletely blocked, a QRS complex will not be observed immediately following the P wave; yet a subsequent P wave may be followed by a narrow QRS complex. In a complete AV block, no communication exists between the atria and the ventricles. As a result, the impulse originating at the SA node travels normally through the atria, but does not progress through the AV node to the ventricles. The ventricles then start initiating ventricular beats at their own inherent rate. In this circumstance, the atria and the ventricles beat independently of each other. In AV blocks, the main differentiating features center on the PR interval, regularity/irregularity of R-R interval and the conduction ratio of P waves to QRS complexes.

FIRST-DEGREE HEART BLOCK

In first-degree heart block (1° HB), the rhythm follows the normal conduction pathway from the SA node through the atria, AV junction, bundle of His, and Purkinje fibers, but the impulse is delayed as it passes through the AV node. The delay is seen on ECG by a prolonged PR interval of greater than 0.20 seconds whose timing is consistent from beat to beat (Fig. 6-1).

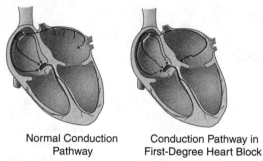

Normal Conduction   Conduction Pathway in
Pathway   First-Degree Heart Block

Figure 6-1   Conduction pathway in first-degree heart block.

First-Degree Heart Block Causes

The rhythm may be seen in healthy individuals, but is more commonly associated with an inferior wall myocardial infarction and medications that slow the conduction time through the AV node. An inferior wall myocardial infarction results from occlusion to the proximal end of the right coronary artery, which leads to damage to the inferior wall, right ventricle, and AV node in most patients. The lack of oxygenated blood flow to the AV node makes the node ischemic and delays the transmission of the electrical impulse from the SA node, resulting in a first-degree heart block. Because of the positive correlation between first-degree heart blocks in inferior wall myocardial infarcted patients and the progression to higher-level AV node blockage, these patients require close monitoring. Both vagal stimulation and medications that may cause bradycardia can slow the electrical conduction time including the PRI.

First-Degree Heart Block Causes

- Vagal stimulation
- Drug-related response
  — Digoxin
  — Beta blockers
  — Calcium channel blockers
  — Amiodarone
  — Procainamide
- Disease-related response
  — Myocardial ischemia/infarction, particularly inferior wall
  — Hyperkalemia

First-Degree Heart Block Assessment

First-degree heart block is typically asymptomatic, but may progress to more serious rhythm disturbances. When listening carefully, the first heart sound may have a diminished strength.

First-Degree Heart Block Interpretation Criteria

In first-degree heart block, the rhythm may be bradycardic, normal rate, or tachycardic; therefore the underlying rhythm must also be interpreted. An example of documentation of this rhythm might be "sinus bradycardia with first-degree heart block (SB with 1° HB)." The three main components of this rhythm are a prolonged constant PR interval, regular R-R interval, and one P wave for each QRS complex (Fig. 6-2).

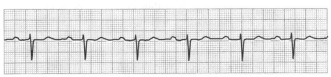

Figure 6-2   First-degree heart block.

First-Degree Heart Block Interpretation Criteria

1. Rhythm: regular
2. Rate: usually 60–100 bpm, but dependent on underlying rhythm
3. P waves: upright, uniform and round in a 1:1 ratio
4. PRI: greater than 0.20 seconds, constant
5. QRS I: less than 0.12 sec

Review Question

What criterion distinguishes this rhythm from NSR?_____

[PRI greater than 0.20 seconds]

First-Degree Heart Block Care Measures

Essentially, treatment for first-degree heart block is centered on monitoring the ECG for progression of the rhythm into a higher degree of heart block. Concurrently, assessing for and treating the possible causes of first-degree heart block can eradicate the prolonged PRI and return the tracing to the patient's underlying rhythm. Consideration of potential causes and their treatments could include measures such as the prevention of vagal stimulation through use of laxatives and antiemetics; discontinuation of causative drugs (digoxin, beta blockers, calcium channel blockers, amiodarone, or procainamide); use of Kayexalate, regular insulin and D_{50}, furosemide, and/or dialysis to treat hyperkalemia; and interventions to treat and prevent the extension of myocardial damage.

First-Degree Heart Block Care Measures

- Carefully monitor the ECG for progression of the rhythm to a higher degree of AV block.
- Treat the cause.

SECOND-DEGREE HEART BLOCK, WENCKEBACH

Second-degree (Wenckebach) heart block is a rhythm characterized by a group of patterned beating where the PRI becomes longer with each successive beat until a QRS is dropped and then the pattern repeats itself. The conduction pathway starts in the SA node and flows through the atria along the normal pathway until it reaches the AV node. At the AV node, the conduction is increasingly delayed until one QRS complex is completely blocked from flowing through the ventricles. In the late 1800s, Karel Wenckebach was one of the first to recognize and document his findings about this rhythm (Mendoza Davila and Varnon, 2008). In 1924, Woldemar Mobitz further analyzed the rhythms identified by Wenckebach as a second-degree heart block into two rhythms which Mobitz classified as Mobitz 1 (Wenckebach) and Mobitz 2 (Silverman et al., 2004). Consequently, the rhythm has previously been known by both names: Wenckebach and Mobitz type 1 second-degree AV block, but today is most commonly called Wenckebach (Fig. 6-3).

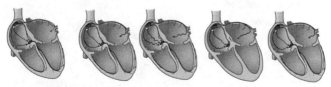

Normal Conduction   Conduction Pathway in Wenckebach
Pathway

Figure 6-3 Conduction pathway in second-degree heart block, Wenckebach.

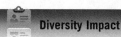
Diversity Impact

Seen in children, especially in the presence of some congenital heart defects such as tetralogy of Fallot. Incidence increases gradually with advancing age.

Wenckebach Causes

Wenckebach may be normal in athletes and children, particularly if their rhythm is slow. Drugs that have a parasympathetic response or slow the heart rate may predispose the patient to Wenckebach. In 90% of the population, the right coronary artery supplies the AV node. An occlusion of the right coronary artery can lead to delays in conduction through the AV node as well as an inferior wall myocardial infarction. Some structural cardiac changes, including tetralogy of Fallot and valvular damage, may affect conduction through the AV node related to the close proximity of the AV node's relationship to these structures. Hyperkalemia may cause the action potential to rise more slowly resulting in a slower conduction of the impulse throughout all areas of the heart including conduction through the AV node leading to an incomplete or complete heart block.

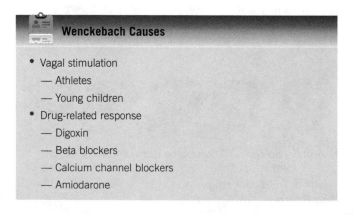
Wenckebach Causes

- Vagal stimulation
  - Athletes
  - Young children
- Drug-related response
  - Digoxin
  - Beta blockers
  - Calcium channel blockers
  - Amiodarone

- Disease-related response
  — Inferior wall myocardial ischemia/infarction
  — Structural heart disease
    ▪ Tetralogy of Fallot
    ▪ Mitral valve disease
  — Hyperkalemia

Wenckebach Assessment

Wenckebach is usually asymptomatic except for an irregular pulse. An irregular pulse occurs due to the delay and occasional complete block of conduction of the beats through the AV node. A reduced cardiac output with its associated signs and symptoms may occur, especially when the ventricular rate drops to less than 45 beats per minute (bpm).

Wenckebach Assessment

- Usually asymptomatic
- Irregular pulse
- Decreased cardiac output
  — Weakness
  — Dizziness
  — Hypotension

Wenckebach Interpretation Criteria

Wenckebach occurs in a pattern of grouped beating, which is the key to interpreting this rhythm. The PRI lengthens with each successive beat until one QRS complex is dropped; and then the pattern begins again, starting with a shorter PRI that progressively lengthens with each successive beat until a QRS complex is dropped. In Wenckebach, the pattern of grouped beating repetitively cycles upon itself until it converts back to the patient's underlying rhythm or evolves into a higher level of AV block. The P waves reflecting atrial contraction are regular, but due to the delay or block of the conduction of the electrical impulse, the QRS waves and ventricular contractions are irregular. The three main components of this rhythm are a lengthening PRI until one QRS complex dropped, irregular R-R interval, and one to two P waves for each QRS complex (Fig. 6-4).

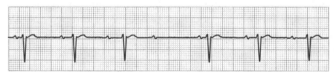

Figure 6-4   Second-degree heart block, Wenckebach.

Wenckebach Interpretation Criteria

1. Rhythm:
   A. Atrial: regular
   B. Ventricular: irregular with a pattern of grouped beating
2. Rate:
   A. Atrial: 60–100 bpm
   B. Ventricular: bradycardic or normal
3. P waves: upright, uniform, and round
4. PRI: lengthening of PRI with successive beats until one QRS complex is dropped
5. QRS I: less than 0.12 sec

Review Question

What criteria distinguishes this rhythm from NSR?_____

[Lengthening of PRI with successive
beats until one QRS complex is dropped;
and then pattern repeats]

Wenckebach Care Measures

Similar to first-degree heart block, Wenckebach is typically asymptomatic. The rhythm is most likely to resolve spontaneously, but may progress to a higher level of blockage in myocardial infarction patients, especially in the first few hours. Per usual, the course of action needs to include treating the cause of the problem such as removing vagal stimulation, discontinuing or decreasing dosages of drug causative agents, and lowering potassium levels. Occasionally, atropine is needed to speed the heart rate up to improve cardiac output, but one needs to be watchful for ventricular dysrhythmias in patients with myocardial ischemia/infarction. Because Wenckebach usually resolves after a few days, the need for pacing is rare.

Wenckebach Care Measures

- Carefully monitor the ECG for progression of the rhythm to a higher degree of AV block.
- Treat the cause.
- For bradycardic symptomatic Wenckebach.
  — Administer atropine.
  — Apply transcutaneous pacemaker.

SECOND-DEGREE HEART BLOCK, MOBITZ 2°

Mobitz 2° is a more rarely seen rhythm than Wenckebach, but dramatically more dangerous due to its propensity to advance to third-degree heart block. When seen, the rhythm is characterized by an intermittent complete block of impulses in the location of the bundle branches. The flow of electrical conduction progresses normally from the SA node through the atrial pathway and AV node. At the bundle branches, the impulse is intermittently blocked, creating a rhythm where two or more P waves are conducted for each QRS. When the P waves are conducted on through the bundle branches, the PRI is constant. Occasionally, a complete block of one of the bundle branches may occur with an intermittent block of the other bundle branch. When this happens, the QRS complex will be wider and longer than 0.12 seconds (Fig. 6-5).

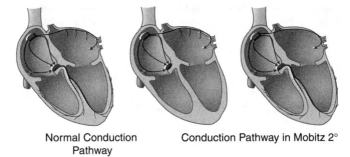

Normal Conduction
Pathway

Conduction Pathway in Mobitz 2°

Figure 6-5   Conduction pathway in second-degree heart block, Mobitz 2°.

Mobitz 2° Causes

The left coronary artery supplies blood flow to the bundle branches. Occlusion of the left coronary artery may produce an anterior wall myocardial infarction with a Mobitz 2° rhythm seen with a wide QRS complex. Occlusion of the right coronary artery is more likely to produce an inferior wall myocardial infarction, with a Mobitz 2° usually seen with a narrower QRS complex.

Mobitz 2° Causes

- Disease-related response
  — Anterior wall or inferior wall myocardial infarction
  — Chronic cardiac disease

Mobitz 2° Assessment

An irregular pulse and bradycardia may occur dependent on the impulse flow through the bundle branches. Even though the rhythm may be asymptomatic, the patient may experience some signs and symptoms of decreased cardiac output due to the lack of ventricular contractions with some of the conducted atrial complexes. Analysis of a 12-lead ECG is critical to determine the site of the infarct. Mobitz 2° in the presence of an inferior wall myocardial infarction is less worrisome than when seen with an anterior wall myocardial infarction. The combination of an anterior wall myocardial infarction and Mobitz 2° rhythm is considered dangerous.

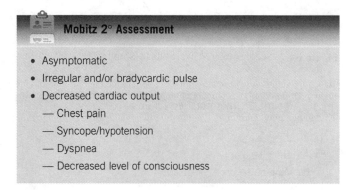

Mobitz 2° Assessment

- Asymptomatic
- Irregular and/or bradycardic pulse
- Decreased cardiac output
  — Chest pain
  — Syncope/hypotension
  — Dyspnea
  — Decreased level of consciousness

Mobitz 2° Interpretation Criteria

The three main components of this rhythm are a constant PRI, usually regular R-R interval, and one or more P waves for each

QRS complex. The PRI is constant whenever the P waves are conducted through to the ventricles generating the QRS complex. Since several of the atrial impulses are not conducted to the ventricles, the ventricular rate varies and is less than the atrial rate, creating a high likelihood of a bradycardic rhythm. Mobitz 2° may be differentiated into a 2:1 block or advanced Mobitz block. The distinction between 2:1 and advanced is the ratio of P waves to QRS. Sometimes, the ventricular response has a variable conduction ratio, which makes the ventricular rhythm irregular. As the number of P waves compared to the number of QRS complexes increases in advanced Mobitz 2°, the amount of block becomes more severe. Keys to distinguish Mobitz 2° from Wenckebach center on evaluation of the PRI and the width of the QRS complex. In Wenckebach, the PRI is typically lengthened with a narrow QRS; while in Mobitz 2°, the PRI is more apt to be normal with a wider QRS. If the rhythm is present in the patient with a myocardial infarction, analysis of a 12-lead ECG is critical to determine if the site of the infarct is anterior or inferior (Fig. 6-6).

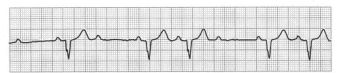

Figure 6-6   Second-degree heart block, Mobitz 2°.

Mobitz 2° Interpretation Criteria

1. Rhythm:
   A. Atrial: regular
   B. Ventricular: usually regular
2. Rate:
   A. Atrial: usually 60–100 bpm
   B. Ventricular: less than atrial rate, frequently bradycardic

3. P waves: upright, uniform, and round with usually more than one P wave for every QRS
4. PRI: constant for conducted P waves, may be prolonged
5. QRS I: occasionally greater than 0.12 sec, absent after some P waves

Review Question

What criteria distinguishes this rhythm from NSR?_____

[Greater than one P wave for every QRS with PRI constant and usually regular R-R intervals]

Mobitz 2° Care Measures

The first step to take is to assess for the signs and symptoms of a reduced cardiac output, which is highly likely with this rhythm. If the patient is asymptomatic, administer oxygen, start an intravenous line, apply transcutaneous pacer pads, and assess for the ability to achieve capture; then place the pacer on standby and call the cardiologist. In the event that the transcutaneous pacer does not capture, begin to prepare the patient for a transvenous pacemaker. When the patient has evidence of a reduced cardiac output, begin transcutaneous pacing, call the cardiologist, and prepare the patient for a transvenous pacemaker.

Mobitz 2° Care Measures

- Assess impact of the rhythm on the patient's clinical signs and symptoms.
- Administer oxygen.
- Insert intravenous catheter.

Asymptomatic
- Attach transcutaneous pacer pads.
- Assess for capture of pacer.
- Place pacer on standby.
- Call the cardiologist.

Symptomatic
- Begin transcutaneous pacing.
- Call the cardiologist.
- Prepare for transvenous pacemaker.

THIRD-DEGREE HEART BLOCK (COMPLETE HEART BLOCK, 3° HB)

Third-degree heart block (complete heart block, or 3° HB) is a life-threatening rhythm! A complete blockage of the transmission of impulses occurs at the AV node, bundle of His or the His–Purkinje system. The SA node initiates beats that conduct through the atria to the AV node, and then the transmission is completely blocked. As a result, the junctional tissue or ventricles start initiating beats at their inherent rates. In this rhythm, the atria and ventricles are beating independently of each other. Third-degree heart block is also known as complete heart block (CHB). See Figure 6-7.

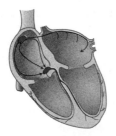
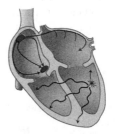

Normal Conduction
Pathway

Conduction Pathway in
Third-Degree Heart Block

Figure 6-7   Conduction pathway in third-degree heart block.

Diversity Impact

Characteristics of congenitally acquired third-degree heart block usually include a junctional escape focus, asymptomatic presentation, and a higher mortality rate as a neonate than in adolescence (Conover, 2003).

Third-Degree Heart Block Causes

Neonates may be born with third-degree heart block or acquire the rhythm as a result of cardiac surgery (Chou & Knilans, 1996). Third-degree heart block is more likely to occur after an inferior wall myocardial infarction than after an anterior wall myocardial infarction. Third-degree heart block as a result of an inferior wall myocardial infarction is more apt to be temporary, lasting a week or so and resolving spontaneously. On the other hand, third-degree heart block from an anterior wall myocardial infarction is more apt to be a permanent rhythm. Third-degree heart block is seen more frequently in patients with type II diabetes mellitus (Movahed et al., 2005).

Third-Degree Heart Block Causes

- Congenital
- Disease-related response
  — Inferior wall myocardial infarction
  — Anterior wall myocardial infarction

Third-Degree Heart Block Assessment

The rhythm is typically symptomatic related to the degree of bradycardia, loss of atrial kick, and the decreased cardiac output. The bradycardia occurs related to the slower inherent rates of the junctional and ventricular tissues when those areas assume pacemaker functions. When the atria and ventricles do not beat in conjunction with each other, a loss of atrial kick occurs and leads to 30% reduction in cardiac output with its associated signs and symptoms.

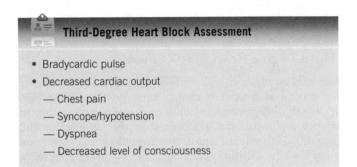

Third-Degree Heart Block Assessment

- Bradycardic pulse
- Decreased cardiac output
  — Chest pain
  — Syncope/hypotension
  — Dyspnea
  — Decreased level of consciousness

Third-Degree Heart Block Interpretation Criteria

A third-degree heart block that evolves from an inferior wall myocardial infarction usually has a junctional escape focus; whereas an anterior wall myocardial infarction is more likely to have a ventricular escape focus. The difference between a junctional escape focus and a ventricular escape focus is the length of the QRS complex interval and the ventricular rate. A junctional escape focus will have a QRS complex interval of less than 0.12 seconds and a typical heart rate of 40 to 60 bpm; while a ventricular focus will have a QRS complex interval of greater than 0.12 seconds and a typical heart rate of 20 to 40 bpm. Because the atria and ventricles are beating independently of each other, no PRI exists due to a lack of relationship between the P wave and the QRS complex. The three main components of this rhythm are what appears to be an inconsistent PRI (in fact, no PRI exists in this rhythm), a regular R-R interval, and no relationship between the number of P waves and the QRS complex (Fig. 6-8).

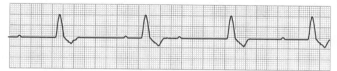

Figure 6-8   Third-degree heart block.

Third-Degree Heart Block Interpretation Criteria

1. Rhythm:
   A. Atrial: regular
   B. Ventricular: regular
2. Rate:
   A. Atrial: usually 60–100 bpm
   B. Ventricular: based on location of pacer site
      i. Junctional: 40–60 bpm
      ii. Ventricular: 20–40 bpm
3. P waves: upright, uniform, and round with no relationship to QRS
4. PRI: none
5. QRS I: based on location of pacer site
   i. Junctional: less than 0.12 sec
   ii. Ventricular: greater than 0.12 sec

Review Question

What criteria distinguishes this rhythm from NSR?_____

[Inconsistent PRI appearance, regular R-R interval, and no relationship between the number of P waves and QRS complexes]

Third-Degree Heart Block Care Measures

As stated before, the first step is to determine the effect of the rhythm on the patient's signs and symptoms. Many times, third-degree heart block from an inferior wall myocardial infarction resolves within a few days and does not need treatment. A transcutaneous pacemaker needs to be available. The recommendation is to attach the transcutaneous pacer pads and check for capture to determine the functioning of the pacer before an emergency strikes. For a patient with third-degree heart block in the presence of an anterior wall myocardial infarction, a transvenous pacemaker is more likely to be required. A transcutaneous pacemaker is used while arrangements for insertion of a transvenous pacemaker are being conducted.

Third Degree Heart Block Care Measures

- Assess impact of the rhythm on the patient's clinical signs and symptoms.
- Administer oxygen.
- Insert intravenous catheter.
- May apply transcutaneous pads and begin pacing.
- May prepare for transvenous pacemaker.

BUNDLE BRANCH BLOCK

In a bundle branch block (BBB), the electrical conduction is completely or incompletely blocked on its pathway down the right or left bundle branches. For a right bundle branch block (RBBB), the electrical impulse is blocked from flowing down the interventricular septum to the right ventricle. As a result, the impulse flows down the left bundle branch to the left ventricle, causing the left ventricle to depolarize and contract before the right ventricle. The right ventricle receives the electrical impulse indirectly from the left ventricle. On the ECG, the longer alternate pathway results in a wider QRS and typically a classic "rabbit-ear" formation of the R waves in leads V_1 and V_2. The right bundle branch is thinner and more frequently damaged than the left bundle branch. For a left bundle branch block (LBBB) to occur, the electrical impulse flows normally through the SA node, atrial pathway, AV node, and bundle of His, but then is blocked from traveling down the left bundle branch. Consequently, the electrical impulse flows down the right bundle branch along the interventricular septum to the right ventricle and then indirectly to the left ventricle. Again, the alternate pathway takes longer, creating a wide QRS and the classic "rabbit-ear" formation of the R waves in leads V_5 and V_6. The V_1 lead is located on the right side of the heart, which is why the classic rabbit ear formation occurs in V_1 and V_2 for an RBBB. The V_5 and V_6 leads are located on the left side of the heart, which is why the rabbit-ear formation occurs in V_5 and V_6 for a left bundle branch block. See Figure 6-9 for RBBB and Figure 6-10 for LBBB.

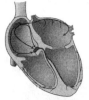 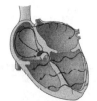

Normal Conduction
Pathway

Conduction Pathway in Right
Bundle Branch Block

Figure 6-9   Conduction pathway in right bundle branch block.

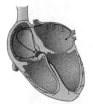

Normal Conduction
Pathway

Conduction Pathway in Left
Bundle Branch Block

Figure 6-10   Conduction pathway in left bundle branch block.

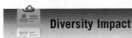

Diversity Impact

May be seen after congenital heart surgery for tetralogy of Fallot, atrial and/or ventricular septal defects, and pulmonary stenosis.

Bundle Branch Block Causes

Due to the structural nature of the right bundle branch being thin, a RBBB may be seen in healthy individuals as well as people with adverse reactions to drugs or disease-related states including myocardial infarctions and coronary artery disease. The structure of the left ventricle is thicker and splits into three offshoots called the septal, anterior, and posterior fascicles. LBBB is considered more serious and in combination with a new myocardial infarction has a higher mortality rate.

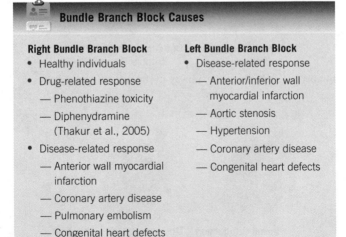

Bundle Branch Block Causes

Right Bundle Branch Block
- Healthy individuals
- Drug-related response
  - Phenothiazine toxicity
  - Diphenydramine (Thakur et al., 2005)
- Disease-related response
  - Anterior wall myocardial infarction
  - Coronary artery disease
  - Pulmonary embolism
  - Congenital heart defects

Left Bundle Branch Block
- Disease-related response
  - Anterior/inferior wall myocardial infarction
  - Aortic stenosis
  - Hypertension
  - Coronary artery disease
  - Congenital heart defects

Bundle Branch Block Assessment

Both right and left bundle branch blocks independent of a myocardial infarction will usually present asymptomatically. Occasionally, patients will experience weakness and dizziness due to a decreased cardiac output if the patient is also bradycardic.

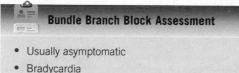

Bundle Branch Block Assessment

- Usually asymptomatic
- Bradycardia
- Weakness
- Dizziness

Bundle Branch Block Interpretation Criteria

Interpretation of bundle branch blocks is more difficult than with the other rhythms discussed so far, due to their multiple variations (left vs. right, anterior vs. posterior, incomplete vs. complete) and similarity to some types of myocardial infarctions. In addition, interpretation of bundle branch blocks requires familiarity with other cardiac leads besides the classic lead II used thus far in this text. The best approach is to compare a previous ECG with the present one to determine the presence of a bundle branch block. The QRS complex is wide, with complete blocks measuring greater than 0.12 seconds. Incomplete blocks may have QRS complexes between 0.10 and 0.11 seconds. Diagnosis of RBBB is determined by a classic pattern of rSR which represents an "M" shape or the commonly called "rabbit ears" in leads V_1 and V_2. In RRBB, the r represents normal depolarization of the interventricular septum, followed by a deep sloping S wave representing normal depolarization of the left ventricle, followed by a tall R wave representing delayed depolarization of the right ventricle. Diagnosis of LBBB is determined by an absent Q wave with a tall sloping R wave, which may or may not be notched in leads I, aVL, V_5, and V_6. The absent Q wave represents a lack of interventricular depolarization between the ventricles, and the sloping R wave demonstrates a delay in left ventricular depolarization. In both RBBB and LBBB, the ST segment is depressed and the T waves are inverted. See Figure 6-11 for RBBB and Figure 6-12 for LBBB.

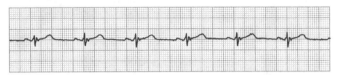

Figure 6-11   Right bundle branch block.

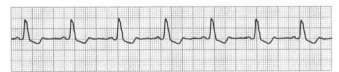

Figure 6-12   Left bundle branch block.

Bundle Branch Block Interpretation Criteria

1. Rhythm: regular
2. Rate: 60–100 bpm, occasional bradycardia
3. P wave: upright, uniform, and round in a 1:1 ratio
4. PRI: 0.12–0.20 sec
5. QRS I: wide, greater than 0.12 sec

Review Questions

What criteria distinguishes RBBB from NSR?_____

[Rabbit-ear formation in V_1 and V_2, wide QRS]

What criteria distinguishes LBBB from NSR?_____

[Absent Q wave with possible rabbit-ear formation
in I, aVL, V_5 and V_6, wide QRS]

Bundle Branch Block Care Measures

Typically, a bundle branch block is asymptomatic. Clarification of the rhythm interpretation usually requires a cardiologist. Care centers around treating the underlying causes such as preventing coronary artery disease and hypertension with lifestyle changes and medications. Reperfusion treatment is recommended for the patient with a LBBB and a new myocardial infarction. When the patient is bradycardic, a transvenous pacemaker may be beneficial to raise the cardiac output by improving the heart rate. Cardiac resynchronization may be used to pace both ventricles of the heart simultaneously optimizing the contracting ability and improving cardiac output.

Bundle Branch Block Care Measures

- Assess impact of the rhythm on the patient's clinical signs and symptoms.
- Treat the cause.
- Reperfusion treatment if in conjunction with new myocardial infarction.
- Transvenous pacemaker if syncopal.
- Cardiac resynchronization for dilated cardiomyopathy and BBB.

PRACTICAL COMPARISON OF ATRIO-VENTRICULAR HEART BLOCKS

Table 6-1 compares the atrioventricular heart block rhythms to each other and to NSR. Areas highlighted in red are features of the rhythm which differentiates the rhythm from Normal Sinus Rhythm.

Table 6-1   Practical Comparison of Atrioventricular Heart Blocks

Distinguishing Features	NSR	1° HB	2° HB, Wenckebach
PRI	0.12–0.20, constant	>0.20 constant	Longer with each beat until QRS complex dropped, pattern repeats
R-R interval	Regular	Regular	Irregular
Conduction ratio of P to QRS complexes	1:1	1:1	1:1 to 2:1
QRS I	<0.12	<0.12	<0.12

2° HB, Mobitz 2	3° HB	RBBB	LBBB
Constant	None	0.12–0.20, constant	0.12–0.20, constant
Regular or irregular	Regular	Regular	Regular
2 or more: 1	No relationship	1:1	1:1
May be >0.12	>0.12	>0.12	>0.12

REFERENCES

Chou TC, Knilans TK. *Electrocardiography in Clinical Practice: Adult and Pediatric.* 4th ed. Philadelphia: Saunders;1996.

Conover M. *Understanding Electrocardiography.* 8th ed. St. Louis: Mosby; 2003.

Mendoza-Davila N, Varnon J, Karel Wenckebach: The story behind the block. *Resuscitation.* Retrieved September 8, 2008, from http://www.sciencedirect.com/science.

Movahed M, Hashemzadeh M, Mazen Jamal M. Increased prevalence of third-degree atrioventricular block in patients with type II diabetes mellitus. *Chest*. 2005;128:2611–2614.

Silverman M, Upshaw CB, Lange HW. Woldemar Mobitz and his 1924 classification of second-degree atrioventricular block. *Circulation*. 2004;110:1162–1167.

Thakur A, Aslam A, Vasavada B, Sacchi T, Khan I. QT interval prolongation in diphenhydramine toxicity. *Int J Cardiol*. 2005;98:341–343.

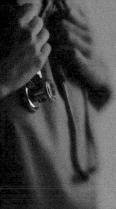

Chapter 7
HELPFUL HINTS TO EASE INTERPRETATION

Once all the possible dysrhythmias have been learned, what do you do when you see a "funky" rhythm on the monitor or ECG? At this point, it's a time for comparison. As discussed previously, it's important to become "boring" when analyzing strips, and approach each strip systematically through the five-step approach. When the answers to the five steps have been obtained, then it's time to compare the rhythms and consider the possible options. Because everyone learns and analyzes information slightly differently, several approaches are presented here. The first method analyzes the strip considering the location site of the rhythm, while the second method analyzes the strip by evaluating a specific distinguishing feature of the rhythm such as extrasystolic beats, bradycardic versus tachycardic rhythms, regular versus irregular rhythms, narrow versus wide QRS I, or pulseless rhythms. Most of the time, one of these features will be readily identifiable and provides a jumping-off point for interpretation. Pick the feature that is most easy for you to figure out; either "funny-looking beats" (extrasystolic beats), rate (bradycardia vs. tachycardia), rhythm (regular vs. irregular), or QRS width (narrow vs. wide). Pulseless rhythms are more easily determined after palpating for a pulse.

DIFFERENTIATION OF RHYTHMS BY LOCATION SITE

At times, deciding which rhythm is presenting itself is easier if one considers the location site precipitating the rhythm. Table 7-1 may assist with differentiating the types of rhythms by location site. Once you have decided on the location site of the rhythm as sinus, atrial, junctional, ventricular, or AV block, compare the characteristics for the rhythms in that location site. You may wish to refer to the Practical Comparison tables at the end of Chapters 2 to 6 for a more complete look at the similarities and differences of the rhythms in each of these groups. Sinus rhythms originating in the sinus node are recognized by upright, round P waves. Sinus rhythms differ among themselves by either rate (bradycardic, normal, or tachycardic) or rhythm (regular or irregular). When the rhythm begins in the atria, a "funny-looking P wave" differing from the patient's sinus node P wave is seen on the ECG. Atrial rhythms differ among themselves in the configuration of the P wave and exhibition of atrial activity and ventricular response rate. The P′ wave or atrial activity may be seen as flattened, notched, inverted P′ waves or P′ waves that vary from the patient's baseline P wave, sawtooth F waves or a chaotic baseline between two R waves. Junctional rhythms may conduct retrogradely back through the atria, creating an inverted P wave that may occur before, after, or hidden inside the QRS. When the P′ wave is found before the QRS, the P′RI is less than 0.12 seconds. Predominantly, junctional rhythms vary between themselves related to the rate of the rhythm or location of the inverted P′ wave. Generally, ventricular rhythms have wide, bizarre QRS waves with prolonged QRS Is of greater than 0.12 seconds. Differences between ventricular rhythms lie in the frequency of the ventricular originating beats, rate of the rhythm, and configuration of the QRS. Incomplete or complete block of conduction of the impulses through the AV node results in AV blocks usually revealed as altered PRIs. Blocks may vary between themselves mostly related to R-R regularity, conduction ratios of P waves to QRS waves, and changes in the PRI.

Table 7-1   Practical Comparison of Rhythms by Location Site

Sinus (upright, uniform, round P waves)
   Normal sinus rhythm
   Sinus bradycardia (<60 bpm)
   Sinus tachycardia (>100 bpm)
   Sinus dysrhythmia (irregular rhythm)
   Sinoatrial arrest (one or more whole PQRST complexes dropped)

Atrial (funny-looking P waves)
   Premature atrial contraction (beat every once in a while)
   Wandering atrial pacemaker (three or more P wave configurations)
   Atrial tachycardia (P wave shape varied from sinus P wave shape, may be obscured into T wave, RVR)
   Atrial flutter (sawtooth flutter pattern, may have RVR)
   Atrial fibrillation (chaotic baseline between R waves, may have RVR, grossly irregular)

Junctional (inverted P wave before, during, after QRS)
   Premature junctional contraction (beat every once in awhile)
   Junctional escape rhythm (40–60 bpm)
   Accelerated junctional rhythm (61–100 bpm)
   Junctional tachycardia (101–180 bpm)
   AV nodal reentrant tachycardia (150–250 bpm)
   AV reentrant tachycardia (150–250 bpm—P at end of QRS or in ST segment)

Ventricular (wide, bizarre QRS)
   Premature ventricular contraction (beat every once in awhile)
   Idioventricular rhythm (20–40 bpm)
   Accelerated idioventricular rhythm (41–100 bpm)
   Ventricular tachycardia (usually regular, 101–250 bpm)
   Ventricular fibrillation (chaotic baseline)
   Asystole (flat line)

AV blocks (PRI)
   First-degree heart block (prolonged constant PRI)
   Second-degree heart block, Wenckebach (lengthening PRI with successive beats until one QRS complex dropped)
   Second-degree heart block, Mobitz 2° (constant PRI with 1 or more P waves per QRS)
   Third-degree heart block (appearance of varying PRI with no relationship between P waves and QRS complexes and one or more P waves per QRS)
   Bundle branch block
      Right bundle branch block (rabbit-ear formation in V_1 and V_2, wide QRS I)
      Left bundle branch block (absent Q wave with possible rabbit-ear formation I, aVL, V_5 and V_6, wide QRS I)

DIFFERENTIATION OF SIMILAR RHYTHM CHARACTERISTICS

Extrasystolic Beats

Extrasystolic beats are extra beats that interrupt the normal rhythm of the heart and occur every once in a while. Extrasystolic beats originate from one of three sites in the heart: the atria (premature atrial contractions [PACs]), junctional tissue (premature junctional contraction [PJCs]), or ventricles (premature ventricular contractions [PVCs]). These rhythms have been previously discussed in Chapters 3, 4, and 5, respectively. The purpose here is to differentiate these extrasystolic beats to ease interpretation. (The areas printed in red in Table 7-2 reflect differences between the extrasystolic beats.) As can be seen in Table 7-2, the main differences that will help to distinguish a PAC from a PJC associated

Table 7-2   Practical Comparison of Extrasystolic Beats

Distinguishing Features	Premature Atrial Contraction (PAC)	Premature Junctional Contraction (PJC)	Premature Ventricular Contraction (PVC)
Rhythm	Irregular when beat occurs	Irregular when beat occurs	Irregular when beat occurs
Rate	Dependent on underlying rhythm	Dependent on underlying rhythm	Dependent on underlying rhythm
P waves	Flattened, notched, or inverted	Inverted before, during, or after QRS	When present, not associated with QRS
PRI	0.12–0.20 sec	When present, less than 0.12 sec	None
QRS I	Less than 0.12 sec	Less than 0.12 sec	Wide, bizarre, and greater than 0.12 sec

with a PVC center on the configuration of the P wave, relationship of P wave to QRS wave (PRI), and the length of time for ventricular depolarization as well as the QRS configuration. Premature atrial contractions and premature junctional contractions can be similar for P wave configuration with inverted P waves; yet the distinguishing feature between these two extrasystolic beats is the length of the PRI. The atrial beats have a PRI between 0.12 and 0.20 seconds, while a junctional beat has a PRI of less than 0.12 seconds. Of the extrasystolic beats, premature ventricular contractions are the beats that have the wide QRS and prolonged QRS I that is not usually seen with either PACs or PJCs. Extrasystolic beats may occur in couplets, salvos, or runs, or in bigeminal, trigeminal, or quadrigeminal patterns particularly for premature atrial contractions and premature ventricular contractions.

Bradycardia Versus Tachycardia

If you have the most confidence with your interpretation of heart rates, then the tables on bradycardia versus tachycardia (Tables 7-3 and 7-4) are a good place to start to decide what the rhythm is that your patient is exhibiting. With both bradycardic and tachycardic rhythms, clinical symptoms evolve from a decrease in cardiac output. Cardiac output equals heart rate multiplied by stroke volume (amount of blood ejected from the heart with each beat). In bradycardia, the lower heart rate reduces the amount of blood that may be ejected from the heart per minute. In tachycardia, the physiologic response may be dependent on age, yet still the faster heart rate may reduce the amount of ventricular filling time, resulting in a lower stroke volume and decreased cardiac output.

Bradycardia

A comparison of the rhythms with slower heart rates or possibly slower heart rates is found in Table 7-3. Bradycardic rhythms may originate from any of the pacer sites within the heart: sinus node, atria, junctional tissue, ventricles, or as conduction disturbance at the AV node. Once the rhythm has been established as being bradycardic, the next step is to compare the remaining characteristics. A rhythm with all normal characteristics would be sinus bradycardia. The absence or dropping of one or more whole

Table 7-3 Practical Comparison of Bradycardic Rhythms

Distin-guishing Features	SB	SA	WAP	JER	IVR
Rhythm	Slightly irregular	Regular, except for dropped PQRST complexes	Slightly irregular	Regular	Usually regular
Rate (bpm)	<60	Usually 60–100, but may vary related to number of dropped PQRST complexes	60–100 or bradycardic	40–60	20–40
P wave	Upright, uniform, round	Upright, uniform, round	Shape varies beat to beat	Inverted before, during, or after QRS	If present, not related to QRS
PRI	0.12–0.20 sec	0.12–0.20 sec	0.12–0.20 sec, varies beat to beat	<0.12 sec when present before QRS	None
QRS I	<0.12 sec	<0.12 sec	<0.12 sec	<0.12 sec	Wide, bizarre, >0.12 sec

SB–Sinus Bradycardia;
SA–Sinoatrial Arrest;
WAP–Wandering Atrial Pacemaker;
JER–Junctional Escape Rhythm;
IVR–Idioventricular Rhythm;
AIVR–Accelerated Idioventricular Rhythm

AIVR	Wencke-bach	Mobitz 2°	3° HB
Regular	Atrial: regular Ventricular: irregular with pattern of grouped beating	Atrial: regular Ventricular: regular or irregular	Regular
41–100	Atrial: 60–100 Ventricular: bradycardic or 60–100	Atrial: 60–100 Ventricular: less than atrial rate, frequently <60	Atrial: 60–100 Ventricular: dependent on pacer site— junctional 40–60; ventricular 20–40
If present, not related to QRS	Upright, uniform, round	Upright, uniform, round; more than one P wave per QRS wave	Upright, uniform, round; no relationship of P wave to QRS wave
None	Lengthening of PRI with successive beats until one QRS complex dropped	Constant, may be prolonged	None
Wide, bizarre, >0.12 sec	<0.12 sec	May be >0.12 sec; absent after some P waves	Dependent on pacer site: junctional <0.12 sec; ventricular >0.12 sec

PQRST complex(es) would be a sinoatrial arrest. An inverted P wave will limit the rhythm choices down to either a wandering atrial pacemaker (WAP) or a junctional escape rhythm—check the PRI to determine which of these two the rhythm is. A WAP will have a PRI between 0.12 and 0.20 seconds while a JER will have a PRI of less than 0.12 seconds when the P wave is before the QRS. A narrow QRS with a pattern of grouped beating due to a lengthening PRI for successive beats until one QRS complex is dropped would be Wenckebach. A wide QRS I of greater than 0.12 seconds will restrict the choices to one of four rhythms: idioventricular (IVR), accelerated idioventricular (AIVR), Mobitz 2°, or third-degree heart block. The next step would be to compare the presence of P waves. Of these four rhythms, only Mobitz 2° has a relationship between the P wave and the QRS complex, where the PRI may be prolonged but is always constant. With IVR, AIVR, and third-degree heart block, the P waves are not associated with the QRS complexes. Differentiate IVR from AIVR by comparing the heart rates. Expect IVR heart rate to be between 20 and 40 bpm compared to AIVR's heart rate of 41 to 100 bpm. In third-degree heart block, the P waves "march" through the rhythm strip appearing exactly where expected despite the ventricular QRS complexes.

Tachycardia

For ease of interpretation of tachycardic rhythms, division of the rhythms into narrow versus wide QRS waves will make the process faster. Rapid heart rates in narrow complex rhythms are referred to as supraventricular tachycardia (SVT). Supraventricular tachycardias originate at or above the AV node. All of the following rhythms may be classified as supraventricular tachycardias: sinus tachycardia, atrial tachycardia, atrial flutter, atrial fibrillation, junctional tachycardia, AV nodal reentrant tachycardia, and AV reentry tachycardia. Due to the nature of the rapidity of the rhythm, many times these rhythms are difficult to differentiate from one another and may simply be called supraventricular tachycardia until the rapid ventricular response is slowed down spontaneously or with therapies such as vagal maneuvers or drugs. This is particularly true when the heart rates are greater than 150 bpm. Once the heart rate drops below 150 bpm, the rhythm may be further diagnosed as originating from a sinus versus atrial versus junctional area related to the characteristics of the P wave and location of the P wave in relationship to the QRS wave. See Figure 7-1.

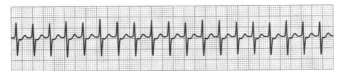

Figure 7-1 Supraventricular tachycardia.

Supraventricular Tachycardia Interpretation Criteria

1. Rhythm: usually regular
2. Rate: 150–250 bpm
3. P wave: configuration similar to sinus P wave or different than sinus P wave located before, during, or after QRS
4. PRI: less than 0.12 sec, 0.12–0.20 sec, or absent
5. QRS I: less than 0.12 sec

In sinus tachycardia, the P wave is upright, uniform and round with a PRI of 0.12 to 0.20 seconds. Three rhythms originating in the atrial tissue vary from sinus tachycardia related to the depiction of atrial activity on the ECG. In atrial tachycardia, the P′ wave varies in shape from the patient's baseline and is frequently obscured into the T wave. In atrial flutter, the P′ waves are actually termed flutter waves and appear on the ECG similar to the edge of a saw or sawtooth waves. Whereas in atrial fibrillation, the atrial activity is so irregularly conducted and so rapidly transmitted that the isoelectric line becomes a chaotic baseline between the R waves. No PRI exists for either atrial flutter or atrial fibrillation. One main distinguishing feature of atrial fibrillation is the grossly irregular nature of the ventricular rhythm. The tachycardic junctional rhythms vary from the sinus and atrial tachycardias due to the presence of an inverted P′ wave before or after the QRS or hidden within the QRS complex. The location of the inverted P′ wave related to the QRS complex assists with distinguishing junctional tachycardia from AV nodal reentrant tachycardia from AV reentrant tachycardia. Junctional tachycardia is typically slower than either AVNRT or AVRT with heart rates of 101 to 180 bpm. In AVNRT, the inverted P′ wave is hidden within or immediately following the QRS complex. In AVRT, the P′ wave moves closer or within the ST segment. Only two tachycardic rhythms exist with a ventricular focus: a wide QRS (ventricular tachycardia) or totally chaotic baseline (ventricular fibrillation). When the heart rates are high, bundle branch block and atrial fibrillation may be misdiagnosed as ventricular tachycardia instead of a supraventricular tachycardia. See Table 7-4.

Regular Versus Irregular

If you have the most confidence with your interpretation of regular and irregular rhythms, then the tables on regular and irregular rhythms (Tables 7-5 and 7-6) are a good place to start to decide what your patient is exhibiting. ECG strips were previously broken into three classifications for rhythm: regular, regularly irregular, and irregularly irregular. The last classification of irregularly irregular has an oxymoronic aspect, contradicting itself, and is now outdated. As a result, the ECG cardiac rhythms discussed in this text are categorized as either regular rhythms or irregular rhythms for ease of interpretation. When reviewing the cardiac rhythms learned, please note that several rhythms may be "usually regular" meaning that at times the rhythm can be irregular. All of the "usually regular" rhythms are represented under regular rhythms, but designated as "usually regular" to increase interpretation ability. Extrasystolic beats (PACs, PJCs, PVCs) discussed above typically cause an irregular rhythm by breaking up the underlying rhythm with a "funny-looking beat," and are differentiated in Table 7-2.

Regular

Regular rhythms exist in all location sites of dysrhythmias and include normal sinus rhythm, sinus bradycardia, sinus tachycardia, atrial tachycardia, atrial flutter, junctional escape rhythm, accelerated junctional rhythm, junctional tachycardia, AV nodal reentrant tachycardia, AV reentrant tachycardia, idioventricular rhythm, accelerated idioventricular rhythm, ventricular tachycardia, first-degree heart block, and third-degree heart block. Once you have established that the rhythm is regular, the next easiest step is to compare the QRS I. The narrow QRS regular rhythms may be differentiated based on their configuration and location of the P wave and the heart rate. Upright, uniform, and round P waves are present in normal sinus rhythm, sinus bradycardia, sinus tachycardia and first-degree heart block. These four rhythms may be compared by rate and PRI. The difference between the three sinus rhythms is based on rate with normal sinus rhythm rate between 60 and 100 bpm, sinus bradycardia rate less than 60 bpm and sinus tachycardia rate between 101 and 180 bpm. In each of these sinus rhythms, the PRI is between 0.12 and 0.20 seconds. First-degree heart block has a constant prolonged PRI of greater than 0.20 seconds. Atrial tachycardia and atrial flutter vary based on the configuration of the P wave or flutter wave. Sawtooth patterns are seen with atrial flutter and the P wave shape varies from the patient's sinus P wave, frequently obscured by the T wave in atrial tachycardia. The junctional rhythms are similar in that the P waves are inverted before, during, or after the QRS complex. Rates vary for junctional rhythms, with junctional escape rhythm at 40 to 60 bpm, accelerated junctional rhythm at 61 to 100 bpm, junctional tachycardia at 101 to 180 bpm, and AV nodal reentrant tachycardia and AV reentrant tachycardia at 150 to 250 bpm. AVNRT and AVRT differ based on the location of the inverted P wave, with the P wave occurring early after the QRS in AVNRT and later or in the ST segment for AVRT.

The only four wide QRS rhythms are idioventricular rhythm, accelerated idioventricular rhythms, ventricular tachycardia, and third-degree heart block. Idioventricular and accelerated idioventricular rhythms may or may not have P waves. If P waves are present, no relationship exists between the P wave and the QRS wave. These two rhythms differ by heart rates: 20 to 40 bpm for idioventricular rhythm and 41 to 100 bpm for accelerated idioventricular rhythm. Ventricular tachycardia has a fast heart rate of 101 to 250 bpm; while third-degree heart block has a normal heart rate or even more likely bradycardia. Third-degree heart block

Table 7-4 Practical Comparison of Tachycardic Rhythms

Distin-guishing Features	ST	AT	A-flutter	AF
Rhythm	Regular	Regular	Usually regular	Grossly irregular
Rate (bpm)	101–180	150–250	Atrial: 240–450 Ventricular: 60–180	60–200
P wave	Upright, uniform, round	Varied shape, may be obscured into T wave	Flutter waves with sawtooth appearance	None
PRI	0.12–0.20 sec	Usually 0.12–0.20 sec	None	None
QRS I	<0.12 sec	Usually <0.12 sec	<0.12 sec	<0.12 sec

ST–Sinus Tachycardia;
AT–Atrial Tachycardia;
A-flutter–Atrial Flutter;
AF–Atrial Fibrillation;
JT–Junctional Tachycardia;
VT–Ventricular Tachycardia;
VF–Ventricular Fibrillation
AVNRT–AV Nodal Reentrant Tachycardia;
AVRT–AV Reentrant Tachycardia

JT	AVNRT	AVRT	VT	VF
Regular	Usually regular	Regular	Usually regular	Chaotic baseline
101–180	150–250	150–250	101–250	Unable to determine
Inverted before, during, or after QRS	Hidden or inverted after the QRS	Inverted at end of QRS or early in ST segment	If present, not related to QRS	None
<0.12 sec when present	None	None	None	None
<0.12 sec	Usually <0.12 sec	Usually <0.12 sec	Wide, bizarre; >0.12 sec	None

Table 7-5 Practical Comparison of Regular Rhythms

Distinguishing Features	NSR	SB	ST	AT	A–Flutter	JER	AJR
Rhythm	Regular	Regular/slightly irregular	Regular	Regular	Atrial: regular Ventricular: regular or irregular	Regular	Regular
Rate (bpm)	60–100	<60	101–180	150–250	Atrial: 240–450 Ventricular: 60–180	40–60	61–100
P Wave	Upright, uniform, round	Upright, uniform, round	Upright, uniform, round	Varied shape, may be obscured into T wave	Flutter with sawtooth appearance	Inverted before, during, or after QRS	Inverted before, during, or after QRS
PRI	0.12–0.20 sec	0.12–0.20 sec	0.12–0.20 sec	Usually 0.12–0.20 sec	Unable to be determined	<0.12 sec when present before QRS	<0.12 sec when present before QRS
QRS I	<0.12 sec	<0.12 sec	<0.12 sec	Usually <0.12 sec	<0.12 sec	<0.12 sec	<0.12 sec

(Continued)

Table 7-5 Practical Comparison of Regular Rhythms (*Continued*)

Distinguishing Features	JT	AVNRT	AVRT	IVR	AIVR	VT	1° HB	3° HB
Rhythm	Regular	Usually regular	Regular	Usually regular	Regular	Usually regular	Regular	Regular
Rate (bpm)	101–180	150–250	150–250	20–40	41–100	101–250	60–100	Atrial: 60–100 Ventricular: dependent on pacer site—junctional 40–60; ventricular 20–40
P Wave	Inverted before, during, or after QRS	Hidden or inverted after the QRS	Inverted at end of QRS or early in ST segment	If present, not related to QRS	If present, not related to QRS	If present, not related to QRS	Upright, uniform, round	Upright, uniform, round; no relationship of P wave to QRS wave
PRI	<0.12 sec when present before QRS	None	None	None	None	None	>0.20 sec, constant	None
QRS	<0.12 sec	Usually <0.12 sec	Usually <0.12 sec	Wide, bizarre; >0.12 sec	Wide, bizarre; >0.12 sec	Wide, bizarre; >0.12 sec	<0.12 sec	Dependent on pacer site: junctional <0.12 sec; ventricular >0.12 sec

has no relationship between the P wave and the QRS wave, creating what appear to be inconstant PRIs.

Please remember that several of the rhythms designated as regular may present with an irregular baseline at times.

Irregular

When an irregular rhythm is seen on ECG, a pulse should also be obtained apically and radially for 1 minute. If the apical and radial pulse is taken simultaneously, a pulse deficit can be determined by subtracting the apical pulse from the radial pulse. Apical pulse – radial pulse = pulse deficit. A pulse deficit informs the practitioner of the number of beats of the heart that are not perfusing the body. Irregular rhythms are seen in sinus, atrial, ventricular, and block rhythms. Notice that junctional rhythms, except for extrasystolic premature junctional contractions, are usually regular rhythms. All of the irregular sinus rhythms have upright, uniform, and round P waves, and may be differentiated from each other by the heart rate. Sinus dysrhythmia has a normal heart rate of 60 to 100 beats per minute and sinoatrial arrest has a lower heart rate than the patient's baseline due to dropping of complete PQRST complexes. Wandering atrial pacemaker differs from the irregular sinus rhythms due to the presence of at least three P-wave configurations. The characteristic that distinguishes Wenckebach from the irregular sinus rhythms is a pattern of the lengthening of the PRI until one QRS complex is dropped with regular P-P intervals and irregular R-R intervals. In an irregular Mobitz 2° rhythm, P waves that are not conducted through to the ventricles lack a pattern of dropped beats that is characteristic of Wenckebach. Another variation between Wenckebach and Mobitz 2° relates to the PRI which varies in Wenckebach and is constant in Mobitz 2°. Although atrial fibrillation and ventricular fibrillation both have chaotic baselines, atrial fibrillation has the chaotic baseline between an irregular pattern of QRS waves while ventricular fibrillation has a completely chaotic baseline with no distinguishable PQRST waves. If the rhythm is grossly irregular with QRS waves, atrial fibrillation is most likely the culprit.

Please remember that several of the rhythms designated as regular may present with an irregular baseline at times. Rhythms

Table 7-6 Practical Comparison of Irregular Rhythms

Distinguishing Features	SD	SA	WAP	AF	Wenckebach	Mobitz 2°	VF
Rhythm	Irregular	Irregular related to dropped PQRST complex	Slightly irregular	Atrial: chaotic baseline Ventricular: grossly irregular	Atrial: regular Ventricular: irregular with grouped beating	Atrial: regular Ventricular: regular or irregular	Chaotic baseline
Rate (bpm)	60–100	Usually 60–100	60–100, bradycardic	Atrial: unable to be determined Ventricular: 60–200	Atrial: 60–100 Ventricular: bradycardic, normal	Atrial: 60–100 Ventricular: less than atrial rate, frequently <60	Unable to determine

(Continued)

Table 7-6 Practical Comparison of Irregular Rhythms (*Continued*)

Distinguishing Features	SD	SA	WAP	AF	Wenckebach	Mobitz 2°	VF
P wave	Upright, uniform, round	Upright, uniform, round	Shape varies beat to beat	None	Upright, uniform, round	Upright, uniform, round; more than one P wave per QRS wave	None
PRI	0.12–0.20 sec	0.12–0.20 sec	0.12–0.20 sec, varies beat to beat	None	Lengthening of PRI with successive beats until one QRS complex dropped	Constant, may be prolonged	None
QRS I	<0.12 sec	<0.12 sec	<0.12 sec	<0.12 sec	<0.12 sec	May be >0.12; absent after some P waves	None

AF—Atrial Fibrillation; 2° HB—second-degree Heart Block; SA—Sinoatrial Arrest; SD—sinus dysrhythmia; VF—Ventricular Fibrillation; WAP—Wondering Atrial Pacemaker.

discussed under regular rhythms which may present with an irregular baseline are sinus bradycardia (SB), atrial flutter, AV nodal reentrant tachycardia, idioventricular rhythm, and ventricular tachycardia (VT).

Narrow Versus Wide QRS

If you have the most confidence with your interpretation of narrow versus wide QRS waves, then the tables on narrow and wide QRS rhythms (Tables 7-7 and 7-8) are a good place to start to decide what your patient is exhibiting. Narrow QRS Is are less than or equal to 0.12 seconds, while wide QRS Is are greater than 0.12 seconds. The rhythms designated below as narrow or wide are based on their usual presentation. Please recognize that some narrow rhythms present with an aberrancy or an alteration in the ventricular conduction pathway that may make the rhythm atypically present with a wider QRS I. QRS Is of greater than 0.12 seconds are more indicative of sudden cardiac death and poorer outcomes; yet is not a predictor of either ventricular tachycardia or ventricular fibrillation (Olshansky, 2005).

Narrow

Narrow QRS waves have a QRS I of less than 0.12 seconds. A narrow QRS wave is formed when the sinus node, atria, or higher junctional tissue is responsible for initiating the beats. In each of these rhythms, the conduction pathway through the ventricles follows the normal depolarization/repolarization route. The variance in these rhythms relates to an issue with the sinus node, atria, or junctional tissue.

Once a narrow QRS wave has been established, comparing the rates of the rhythm is probably the next easiest step. Rhythms with possible rates of less than 60 bpm include sinus bradycardia, wandering atrial pacemaker, junctional escape rhythm, Wenckebach, and Mobitz 2°. These rhythms are distinct from each other by assessing the P wave and PRI. Sinus bradycardia has all the normal characteristics on an ECG except for the heart rate being slow at less than 60 bpm. In a wandering

Table 7-7 Practical Comparison of Narrow QRS Rhythms

Distinguishing Features	NSR	SB	ST	SD	SA	WAP	AT	A-Fluter
Rhythm	Regular	Regular, slightly irregular	Regular	Irregular	Regular except for dropped PQRST complexes	Slightly irregular	Regular	Usually regular
Rate (bpm)	60–100	<60	>100	60–100	Usually 60–100, but may vary related to number of dropped complexes	60–100 or bradycardic	150–250	Atrial: 240–450 Ventricular: 60–180
P wave	Upright, uniform, round	Upright, uniform, round	Upright, uniform, round	Upright, uniform, round	Upright, uniform, round	Shape varies beat to beat	Varied shape, may be obscured into T wave	Flutter waves with sawtooth appearance
PRI	0.12–0.20 sec	0.12–0.20 sec	0.12–0.20 sec	0.12–0.20 sec	0.12–0.20 sec	0.12–0.20 sec, varies beat to beat	Usually 0.12–0.20 sec	Unable to be determined
QRS I	<0.12 sec	<0.12 sec	<0.12 sec	<0.12 sec	<0.12 sec	<0.12 sec	Usually <0.12 sec	<0.12 sec

(Continued)

Table 7-7 Practical Comparison of Narrow QRS Rhythms (*Continued*)

	AF	JER	AJR	JT	AVNRT	AVRT	1° HB	Wenckebach	Mobitz 2°
	Grossly irregular	Regular	Regular	Regular	Usually regular	Regular	Regular	Atrial: regular Ventricular: irregular with grouped beating	Atrial: regular Ventricular: regular or irregular
	60–200	40–60	61–100	101–180	150–250	150–250	60–100	Atrial: 60–100 Ventricular: bradycardic, normal	Atrial: 60–100 Ventricular: less than atrial rate, frequently <60
	None	Inverted before, during, or after QRS	Inverted before, during, or after QRS	Inverted before, during, or after QRS	Hidden or inverted shortly after QRS	Inverted at end of QRS or early in ST segment	Upright, uniform, round	Upright, uniform, round	Upright, uniform, round; more than one P wave per QRS wave
	None	<0.12 sec when present before QRS	<0.12 sec when present before QRS	<0.12 sec when present before QRS	None	None	>0.20 sec	Lengthening of PRI with successive beats until one QRS complex dropped	Constant, may be prolonged
	<0.12 sec	<0.12 sec	<0.12 sec	<0.12 sec	Usually <0.12 sec	Usually <0.12 sec	<0.12 sec	<0.12 sec	<0.12 sec

See Tables 7-5 and 7-6.

Table 7-8   Practical Comparison of Wide QRS Rhythms

Distinguishing Features	IVR	AIVR	VT
Rhythm	Usually regular	Regular	Usually regular
Rate (bpm)	20–40	41–100	101–250
P wave	If present, not related to QRS	If present, not related to QRS	If present, not related to QRS
PRI	None	None	None
QRS I	Wide, bizarre, >0.12 sec	Wide, bizarre, >0.12 sec	Wide, bizarre, >0.12 sec

atrial pacemaker, the shape of the P wave changes from beat to beat. Junctional escape rhythms have inverted P waves before, during, or after the QRS. Wenckebach and Mobitz 2° have one or more P waves to each QRS complex. In Wenckebach, the PRI progressively lengthens with each successive beat until a QRS complex is blocked; yet in Mobitz 2° the PRI is constant with a normal P wave to QRS complex and occasional P waves with blocked QRS complexes.

Narrow QRS waves with heart rates greater than 100 bpm include sinus tachycardia, atrial tachycardia, atrial flutter, atrial fibrillation, junctional tachycardia, AV nodal reentrant tachycardia, and AV reentrant tachycardia. When the heart rate exceeds

VF	3° HB	RBBB	LBBB
Chaotic baseline	Regular	Regular	Regular
Unable to determine	Atrial: 60–100 Ventricular: 20–40	60–100	60–100
None	If present, not related to QRS	Upright, uniform, round, related to QRS	Upright, uniform, round, related to QRS
None	None	0.12–0.20 sec	0.12–0.20 sec
None	None for ventricular focus	None	None

150 bpm, differentiation between the rhythms becomes difficult since the P wave may be obscured due to the rapidity of the heart rhythm. When the heart rate is slowed spontaneously or with vagal maneuvers or drugs, then interpretation is able to be accomplished. See "Tachycardia" earlier in the chapter.

Narrow QRS waves with heart rates between 60 and 100 bpm include normal sinus rhythm, sinus dysrhythmia, sinoatrial arrest, wandering atrial pacemaker, atrial flutter, atrial fibrillation, accelerated junctional rhythm, first-degree AV block, Wenckebach, and Mobitz 2°. These rhythms are distinct from each other by assessing the P wave, PRI, and for irregularity. In the sinus rhythms, the P wave is upright, uniform, and round.

The sinus rhythms may be distinguished from each other based on presence/absence of PQRST complexes or pattern of irregularity. Normal sinus rhythm is a regular rhythm. In sinoatrial arrest, the rhythm is irregular related to the dropping of complete PQRST complexes, while in sinus dysrhythmia, the rhythm is irregular with all PQRST complexes present. The atrial rhythms vary based on the configuration of the P wave. The changes in the shape of the P wave are three varying configurations for wandering atrial pacemaker, sawtooth appearance for atrial flutter, and a chaotic baseline between the R-R intervals for atrial fibrillation. Accelerated junctional rhythm is the only narrow QRS complex ECG strip with inverted P waves before, during, or after the QRS and a PRI of less than 0.12 seconds when located before the QRS complex. In the AV conduction blocks, the P waves are upright, uniform, and round; yet the number of P waves to QRS waves exceeds the one-to-one ratio. Wenckebach has a lengthening PRI with each successive beat until a QRS complex is dropped, creating a two-to-one ratio of P waves to QRS waves for that beat. Mobitz 2° has a normal P wave to QRS complex ratio with a constant PRI except when a QRS complex is dropped.

Wide

Wide QRS waves have a QRS I of greater than 0.12 seconds. A wide QRS I is formed when the ventricles assume automaticity for the heart and initiate beats. In each of these rhythms, P waves, when present, have no relationship to the QRS wave. When a wide QRS is encountered, the first step is to assess if the rhythm is a chronic issue or a new one, and to determine if the rhythm is creating clinical instability within the patient. Clinical instability may be exhibited by palpitations, chest pain, shortness of breath, loss of consciousness, and changes in vital signs.

A new wide complex rhythm with clinical instability needs to be considered a medical emergency until the rhythm is determined to be a chronic state. A new wide complex rhythm may be an aberrantly conducted rhythm or a ventricular rhythm. A chronic rhythm with a QRS I of greater than 0.12 seconds is typically a bundle branch block. Comparing the rhythm to the patient's previous ECGs can be helpful to establish a change in the patient's baseline.

Idioventricular rhythm, accelerated idioventricular rhythm, and ventricular tachycardia differ by the heart rates. With each of these rhythms, the heart rate is faster than in the previous rhythm such as idioventricular rhythm beats at 20 to 40 bpm, accelerated idioventricular rhythm beats at 41 to 100 bpm and ventricular tachycardia beats at 101 to 250 bpm.Ventricular fibrillation has a chaotic baseline with electrical activity that is not portrayed as a QRS wave and is not measurable. All of the wide QRS rhythms are classified as ventricular rhythms except for third-degree heart block. Third-degree heart block is a complete block of the transmission of impulses at the AV node, resulting in the atria and ventricles beating independently of each other. Third-degree heart block is distinguishable from the other wide QRS rhythms because of the marching of the P waves in a regular pattern with no correlation to the ventricular beats.

Pulseless Rhythms

A machine is one of many tools used in determining a patient's problem and should always be used in conjunction with history-taking and physical assessment of the patient. In this case, palpation of pulses is critical. Pulseless rhythms are always considered cardiac arrest and a life-threatening event. Rhythms that do not produce a pulse include sustained ventricular tachycardia, ventricular fibrillation, aystole, and pulseless electrical activity. Differentiation of VT, VF, and asystole can be seen in Table 7-9. In each of these rhythms, P waves are either absent or unrelated to the QRS. The lack of coordination or complete absence of ventricular depolarization leads to a wide, wavy QRS pattern (ventricular tachycardia) to chaotic baseline (ventricular fibrillation) or to a flatline (asystole). As discussed in Chapter 5, pulseless electrical activity may be represented on an ECG as a narrow or wide QRS complex with either a slow or rapid rate such as ST, SVT, or IVR/AIVR, but without a palpable pulse.

Table 7-9 Practical Comparison of Pulseless Rhythms

Distinguishing Features	Ventricular Tachycardia	Ventricular Fibrillation	Asystole
Rhythm	Usually regular	Chaotic baseline	None
Rate	101–250 bpm	Unable to determine	None
P wave	If present, not related to QRS	None	None
PRI	None	None	None
QRS I	Wide, bizarre; >0.12 sec	None	None

A lack of a pulse in each of these rhythms is the critical ingredient for diagnosing pulseless electrical activity. For care of any pulseless rhythm, following the Pulseless Arrest algorithm suggested by the American Heart Association is recommended (see Appendix C).

REFERENCE

Olshansky B. Wide QRS, narrow QRS: what's the difference? *J Am Coll Cardiol*. 2005;46:317–319.

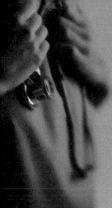

Chapter 8
ELECTROLYTE ECG CHANGES

POTASSIUM

Serum potassium levels are usually considered to be between 3.5 and 5.0 mEq/L. Potassium is a positively charged ion located predominantly within the intracellular spaces (98%), with the remaining 2% found in the extracellular spaces. Serum potassium levels do not necessarily reflect the total body potassium levels because the principal concentration of potassium is located within the cell. Small changes in potassium levels can have a significant clinical effect on the patient related to the tight normal serum range of 3.5 to 5.0 mEq/L. Potassium fluctuates due to the sodium–potassium pump, gastrointestinal intake, and renal/gastrointestinal excretion. Potassium channel openings are responsible for the resting time or refractory period. Consequently, a low serum potassium level causes the heart to become excitable, while an elevated serum potassium level causes the heart to become slow, with delays or complete blockage of impulses.

Hypokalemia

Hypokalemia is described as a serum potassium level of less than 3.5 mEq/L. In some clinical situations, potassium levels of less than 4.0 or 4.3 mEq/L are considered to be hypokalemic and require treatment. Incidence of hypokalemia is approximately 20% in hospitalized patients and may be up to 14% in clinic patients (Garth, 2007). Hypokalemia increases the rate of cardiac cell depolarization, leading to excitable cells and an inability to open the channels that usually terminate the action potential resulting in the development of extrasystolic beats.

Hypokalemia Causes

Hypokalemia is most frequently caused by loop or thiazide diuretics, which are frequently used to treat chronic heart failure, liver failure, renal failure, and hypertension. A second main cause is related to diarrhea, which accounts for millions of infant deaths particularly in low economic areas of Asia and Africa and is a leading cause of infant death in the United States. Approximately one-half of alcoholic patients hospitalized for withdrawal experience hypokalemia due to inadequate dietary intake and gastric losses from vomiting and diarrhea. Inadequate potassium intake has also lately been observed in post-bariatric surgery patients (Al-Momen and El-Mogey, 2005). Besides inadequate intake and the loss of potassium either via urine or gastrointestinal sources, potassium may also move intracellularly, decreasing the amounts in the vascular system available for muscle function. An example is the administration of regular insulin in patients with diabetes mellitus. The movement of glucose and insulin into the cell draws potassium across the cell membrane, decreasing the serum potassium levels. Alkalotic states may also cause potassium to move from the extracellular to intracellular space. In alkalosis, hydrogen ions move out of the cell in an attempt to regulate the pH. When hydrogen ions move out of the cell, potassium ions move into the cell to replace the positively charged ions.

Hypokalemia Causes

- Therapy-related response
  - — Long-term or high-dose loop or thiazide diuretics
  - — Insufficient amount of potassium in diet
  - — Lack of potassium replacement in IV or TPN
  - — Intravenous insulin therapy without potassium replacement in diabetes mellitus
  - — Adverse effect of beta-adrenergic stimulators

- Disease-related response
  — Gastric losses
    ▪ Vomiting
    ▪ Diarrhea
    ▪ Nasogastric suctioning
  — Alkalosis
  — Alcoholism
  — Postoperative bariatric surgery (Al-Momen and El-Mogey, 2005)
  — Cushing syndrome

Diversity Impact

Hypokalemia is more frequently seen in African Americans than Caucasian Americans who take diuretics—possibly due to a lower potassium dietary intake (Fang et al., 2000).

Hypokalemia Assessment

Because of the action of the electrolyte throughout the body on muscle and nerve function, a depletion of potassium creates an effect on several tissues/organs besides the heart. Signs and symptoms typically start to be observed when the serum potassium level drops below 3.0 mEq/L. For moderate hypokalemia, the patient may experience weakness from the decrease of potassium in the extracellular space, which is needed for skeletal muscle contraction. The effect of hypokalemia on smooth muscle cells is to cause nausea, vomiting, and constipation. As the hypokalemia becomes severe, with serum levels of less than 2.5 mEq/L, the degree of hypotonicity of muscle cells progresses to severe weakness, paralysis, and respiratory failure.

Hypokalemia Assessment

Mild	Moderate	Severe
3.0–4.0 mEq/L	2.5–3.0 mEq/L	<2.5 mEq/L
No symptoms	Palpitations	Severe weakness
	Confusion	Flaccid paralysis
	Weakness	Respiratory failure
	Nausea, vomiting, constipation	Cardiac dysrhythmias
	ECG changes	• PAC
	• U wave	• AF
	• Depressed ST segment	• PVC
	• Flattened T wave	• VT
		• VF

Hypokalemia Interpretation Criteria

As the potassium level starts to decline the ECG may show a U wave, depressed ST segment and/or a flattened T wave. A U wave is a positive deflection in lead II located between the T wave and the P wave. A depressed ST segment is a negative deflection below the isoelectric line located between the S wave and the T wave. Dysrhythmias that may evolve as the serum potassium level continues to drop include premature atrial contractions (PACs), atrial fibrillation (AF), premature ventricular contractions (PVCs), and ventricular tachycardia/fibrillation (VT/VF). The rhythm may become either tachycardic or bradycardic (Fig. 8.1).

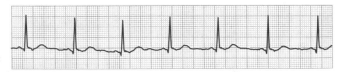

Figure 8-1   Hypokalemia.

Hypokalemia Interpretation Criteria

1. Rhythm: usually regular
2. Rate: 60–100 bpm, may be bradycardic or tachycardic
3. P wave: upright, uniform, and round
4. PRI: 0.12–0.20 sec
5. QRS I: less than 0.12 sec
6. Other: discernible U wave, depressed ST segment and flat
   T wave

Hypokalemia Care Measures

Assessment of the clinical signs and symptoms and ECG changes commensurate with the serum potassium level is the first step when treating hypokalemia. Intake of foods high in potassium is generally sufficient to raise the serum level. Foods high in potassium content include oranges, bananas, figs, potatoes, and tomatoes. Oral supplementation is usually needed with the administration of loop and thiazide diuretics. For patients who are asymptomatic with serum potassium levels between 2.5 and 3.5 mEq/L, oral administration of potassium is usually sufficient. Before administering potassium supplements (oral or parenteral), evaluation of renal function through assessment of urinary output and BUN/creatnine levels is critical to avoid the potential for placing the patient in hyperkalemia. Administration of oral potassium supplements of 1 mEq/kg may be expected to raise the serum potassium level by 1 mEq/L 1 hour from ingestion. Oral potassium supplementation needs to be administered with water to decrease the gastric adverse effects. The presence of ECG changes, more severe clinical symptoms, and a cardiac history usually requires intravenous administration of potassium. Intravenous administration of potassium requires an intravenous pump, a two-RN verification of the five rights of drug administration, frequent intravenous site evaluation for infiltration, and a gentle mixing of the intravenous bag prior to hanging to disperse the potassium evenly throughout the intravenous bag. When available, a central line is preferable to a peripheral intravenous catheter for potassium infusions. Cardiac telemetry monitoring is necessary for intravenous potassium administration of 10 mEq/hr. Administration of intravenous potassium supplement of 0.5 mEq/kg infused over 1 hour may be expected to raise the serum potassium level by 0.6 mEq/kg upon completion of the intravenous minibag. Potassium is **never** to be administered via an intravenous push method. To determine outcome, reassess serum potassium level every 1 to 3 hours when infusing intravenous potassium. Serum potassium levels need to be checked after every 60 mEq of intravenous potassium that is administered to the patient. Frequently with more moderate to severe hypokalemia, magnesium will also need to be replaced concurrently or prior to potassium replacement to promote the conservation of potassium by the kidneys. Besides potassium replacement, assessment and treatment of the original cause of the hypokalemia assists in preventing a recurrence of the problem, such as administration of antiemetics and antidiarrheals, possibly adding a potassium-sparing diuretic or an ACE inhibitor to the regimen for hypertension, reducing alcohol intake and withdrawal risk, and maintaining glucose control for patients with diabetes mellitus.

Hypokalemia Care Measures

- Assess impact of the rhythm on the patient's clinical signs and symptoms.
- Assess amount of urinary output and renal function (BUN and creatnine levels).
- Encourage intake of foods high in potassium.
- Usually administer oral potassium chloride 40–80 mEq/day in divided doses for hypokalemia for serum potassium levels between 2.5 and 3.5 mEq/L.

- Usually administer intravenous potassium chloride for potassium levels less than 2.5 mEq/L.
- Assess serum magnesium levels and replace as needed.
- Treat the cause.

 Clinical Alert
Before administering intravenous potassium chloride at 10 mEq/L/hr, place the patient on cardiac monitor and infuse on an intravenous pump. Overdose of intravenous potassium may cause ventricular tachycardia/ fibrillation, leading to asystole.

Hyperkalemia

Hyperkalemia is described as a serum potassium of greater than 5.0 mEq/L. Incidence of hyperkalemia is between 1% and 10% in hospitalized patients (Lederer, 2009). Higher serum potassium levels cause the action potential to rise more slowly, resulting in a slower conduction of the impulse throughout all areas of the heart, which may lead eventually to third-degree heart block. Cardiac cells may depolarize, but be unable to repolarize, creating an asystolic state with a lack of muscle contraction.

Hyperkalemia Causes

Fairly common, temporary increases in potassium may be found in patients who ingest high quantities of potassium-rich foods, use salt substitutes, or are infused with either too large amounts of potassium supplements or have these supplements administered at too rapid a rate. Several medications are also linked to hyperkalemia as an adverse effect, usually as a result of the medication's effect on the hormones in the kidney; these include ACE inhibitors, angiotension II blocking agents, nonsteroidal anti-inflammatory drugs, and potassium-sparing diuretics. Beta blockers may cause an elevation of potassium in the extracellular spaces by blocking the shift of potassium into the cells from beta adrenergic stimulation. Since 90% of potassium excretion occurs via the kidneys, renal failure or renal obstruction may interfere with the excretion of potassium and lead to hyperkalemia. After the administration of multiple units of packed red blood cells and after an incident of trauma or burns, the patient's serum potassium level may rise related to the destruction of cells and leakage of potassium from inside the cells into the extracellular spaces. In acidosis, the hydrogen ion moves into the cell in an attempt to regulate the pH. When hydrogen ions move into the cell, potassium ions move out of the cell to replace the positively charged ions in the extracellular fluid. Thus, in acidosis, patients can often have hyperkalemia. In patients with diabetes mellitus, a two-pronged effect may cause an elevated serum potassium level: acidosis effect and the high glucose in the extracellular space. When insulin is present in sufficient quantities, glucose, insulin, and potassium can move into the cells. The lack of insulin prevents the movement of glucose and potassium into the cell, causing an elevated serum potassium level extracellularly when the glucose level is elevated. Toad venom ingestion has been found mostly in Southeast Asia and China, where the substance has been used as a folk remedy to strengthen the heart. Besides causing a digoxin toxicity effect, toad venom ingestion also creates hyperkalemia in patients (Cheng et al., 2006).

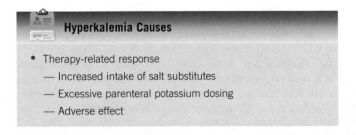

Hyperkalemia Causes

- Therapy-related response
  — Increased intake of salt substitutes
  — Excessive parenteral potassium dosing
  — Adverse effect

- ACE inhibitors
- NSAIDs
- Potassium sparing diuretics—spironolactone
- Beta blockers
- Disease-related response
  - Renal failure/renal obstruction
  - Trauma/burns
  - Diabetic ketoacidosis
  - Acidosis
  - Toad venom ingestion (Cheng et al., 2006)

Diversity Impact

Southeast Asia and China have noted an increased risk for hyperkalemia related to a folk remedy practice of toad venom ingestion taken to strengthen the heart (Cheng et al., 2006). Premature infants and the elderly have a higher incidence of hyperkalemia related to decreased glomerular filtration rates.

Hyperkalemia Assessment

Frequently, in the earlier stages of hyperkalemia, patients are asymptomatic. Unlike hypokalemia, symptoms may not correlate with serum lab values consistently. Patients with chronically elevated serum potassium levels may be asymptomatic, while patients with a rapidly elevated potassium may experience multiple symptoms. Most of the time, signs and symptoms appear after the serum potassium level reaches 7.0 mEq/L, although with a rapid rise the symptoms could appear earlier. Serum potassium levels of greater than 6.0 mEq/L or elevated levels in patients with ECG changes are considered to be clinically significant.

Hyperkalemia Lab Values

Mild	Moderate	Severe
5.1–6.0 mEq/L	6.1–7.0 mEq/L	>7.0 mEq/L

Hyperkalemia Assessment

- Asymptomatic
- Irregular pulse/ECG changes
  — Flat or absent P wave
  — PRI greater than 0.20 sec
  — QRS I greater than 0.12 sec
  — Flat/depressed ST segment
  — Short QT interval
  — Tall tented T wave
  — Bradycardia
  — Bundle branch block
  — Third-degree heart block
- Weakness
- Dyspnea
- Paralysis

Hyperkalemia Interpretation Criteria

When distinguishing between T-wave changes found in myocardial infarctions versus hyperkalemia, the tall, tented T-waves in hyperkalemia are observed in all 12 leads while with a myocardial infarction the changes are only located in leads associated with the site of infarction. Changes to the T wave, making it become more tented with concave sides, are usually the earliest signs of the development of hyperkalemia occurring with serum potassium levels of greater than 5.5 mEq/L. The tall, tented T-wave changes happen in about one-fourth of patients, with the remaining patients demonstrating wide, peaked, tall, or narrow waves. At times, the only ECG change to occur is bradycradia. The next ECG changes to be seen are short QT intervals and depressed ST segments. As serum levels become higher, the PRI becomes prolonged and may advance to bundle branch blocks and then third-degree heart block. When not treated, the rhythm disintegrates into ventricular tachycardia/fibrillation and eventually asystole (Fig. 8-2).

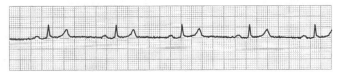

Figure 8-2   Hyperkalemia.

Hyperkalemia Interpretation Criteria

1. Rhythm: regular
2. Rate: 60–100 bpm or bradycardic
3. P wave: flat or absent P wave
4. PRI: greater than 0.20 sec
5. QRS I: greater than 0.12 sec
6. Other: short QT interval, flat/depressed ST segment, and tall, tented T wave

Hyperkalemia Care Measures

Again the first step is to assess the effect on the patient in conjunction with drawing a serum potassium level. When possible, treating the cause through lowering dietary intake of potassium-rich foods to 2 g/day, and discontinuing drugs that cause a rise in potassium, are the beginning steps. In addition, mechanisms that either excrete potassium from the body or move the potassium back into the cells are employed to lower the serum potassium level. Excretion methods include promoting urinary excretion via administration of loop and/or thiazide diuretics and increasing fecal excretion via administration of cation-exchange resins (Kayexalate). Kayexalate is quite effective and may decrease the serum potassium level by 2 mEq/L with one enema. Movement of potassium into the cells may be accomplished by administering 50% dextrose and regular insulin IV. Two other, less-used techniques for moving potassium back into the cells are the administration of sodium bicarbonate, which creates an alkalotic environment and pulls the potassium back into the cells; or the administration of albuterol or epinephrine, which can also drive potassium back into the cells. In more severe cases, intravenous calcium may be given to stabilize the cardiac tissues. Hemodialysis may be performed in more severe cases or in the presence of renal failure. Be careful of overcorrection causing the patient to become hypokalemic. See Table 8-1.

Hyperkalemia Care Measures

* Assess impact of the rhythm on the patient's clinical signs and symptoms.
* Encourage intake of foods low in potassium.
* Discontinue drugs that raise the serum potassium level.
* Administer loop or thiazide diuretics.
* Administer dextrose 50% and regular insulin intravenously
* Administer cation-exchange resin.
* Administer sodium bicarbonate.
* Administer albuterol or epinephrine.
* Administer intravenous calcium.
* Perform hemodialysis.

Table 8-1 Medications Used in Treatment of Acute Hyperkalemia

Medication*	Dosage	Onset	Length of effect	Mechanism of action	Cautions
Calcium gluconate	10 to 20 mL of 10% solution IV over 2 to 3 min	Immediate	30 min	Protects myocardium from toxic effects of calcium; no effect on serum potassium level	Can worsen digoxin toxicity
Insulin	Regular insulin 10 units IV with 50 mL of 50% glucose	15–30 min	2–6 hr	Shifts potassium out of the vascular space and into the cells; no effect on total body potassium	Consider 5% dextrose solution infusion at 100 mL/hr to prevent hypoglycemia with repeated doses. Glucose unnecessary if blood sugar elevated above 250 mg/dL (13.9 mmol/L)
Albuterol (Ventolin)	10 to 20 mg by nebulizer over 10 min (use concentrated form, 5 mg/mL)	15–30 min	2–3 hr	Shifts potassium into the cells, additive to the effect of insulin; no effect on total body potassium	May cause a brief initial rise in serum potassium

(Continued)

Table 8-1 Medications Used in Treatment of Acute Hyperkalemia (*Continued*)

Medication*	Dosage	Onset	Length of effect	Mechanism of action	Cautions
Furosemide (Lasix)	20 to 40 mg IV, give with saline if volume depletion is a concern	15 min to 1 hr	4 hr	Increases renal excretion of potassium	Only effective if adequate renal response to loop diuretic
Sodium polystyrene sulfonate (Kayexalate)	Oral: 50 g in 30 mL of sorbitol solution Rectal: 50 g in a retention enema	1 to 2 hr (rectal route is faster)	4–6 hr	Removes potassium from the gut in exchange for sodium	Sorbitol may be associated with bowel necrosis. May lead to sodium retention

IV = intravenously.

*Medications listed in order of use from most to least urgent.

Adapted or reprinted with permission from *Hyperkalemia*, January 15, 2006. Copyright © 2006 American Academy of Family Physicians. All Rights Reserved.

MAGNESIUM

Serum magnesium levels are usually considered to be between 1.8 and 2.3 mg/dL, or 1.5 and 2.0 mEq/L. Magnesium is a positively charged ion located in the bone (67%), in the intracellular spaces (31%), and in the extracellular spaces (1%) (Novello and Blumstein, 2007). Magnesium levels fluctuate based on the amount absorbed from the ileum in the small intestine and the amount excreted via the large intestine and the kidneys. The kidneys at the proximal tubule and ascending loop of Henle are primarily responsible for the elimination of magnesium. Because magnesium binds to albumin, serum magnesium levels may not be reliable indicators of the total body magnesium level. New intracellular measures and mouth swabbing are currently being examined as more accurate measurements of magnesium levels. Recently, increased interest has been focused on this particular electrolyte and its importance to cardiac functioning. Magnesium acts within the cardiac tissue by blocking calcium entering the calcium channels during the third phase of the action potential and affecting the influx of potassium intracellularly. Consequently, a low serum magnesium level causes the heart to become excitable, while an elevated serum magnesium level causes the heart to become slow with delays or complete blockage of impulses.

Hypomagnesemia

Hypomagnesemia is described as a serum magnesium level of less than 1.8 mg/dL or 1.5 mEq/L. Low magnesium levels reduce the intracellular potassium influx, leading to the development of reentrant circuits causing rhythms such as atrial tachycardias and atrial fibrillation. With low serum magnesium levels, a delay in ventricular repolarization has been identified, which increases the risk for ventricular dysrhythmias.

Diversity Impact

Magnesium levels in obstetric patients may need to be higher to control seizures associated with eclampsia; possibly as high as 3 to 6 mg/100 mL or 2.5 to 5.0 mEq/L.

Hypomagnesemia Causes

In the United States, the most common cause of hypomagnesemia is high alcohol intake, which leads to a reduced dietary intake, increased magnesium excretion renally, and intestinal malabsorption. Thiazide and loop diuretics decrease the renal threshold for reabsorption of magnesium, leading to increased excretion. Cisplatin chemotherapy and aminoglycosides cause magnesium wasting by the kidneys. Starvation and malabsorption cause hypomagnesemia from decreased intake. Acute pancreatitis may present with hypomagnesemia, because magnesium deposits in necrotic areas. When catecholamines stimulate beta receptor sites, magnesium shifts into the cells, lowering the serum magnesium levels. An increased release of catecholamines is believed to be one of the reasons for hypomagnesemia in patients after open heart surgery and in heart failure.

 Hypomagnesemia Causes

* Substance-related response
    — Lack of magnesium replacement in IV or TPN
    — Alcohol
    — Long-term or high-dose loop or thiazide diuretics
    — Cisplatin chemotherapy and aminoglycosides
    — High catecholamine response
* Disease-related response

— Malabsorption

— Diarrhea

— Acute pancreatitis

Hypomagnesemia Assessment

The signs and symptoms of hypomagnesemia are not closely corre-lated to the magnesium level. Hypokalemia and hypomagnesemia frequently occur simultaneously. A low intracellular magnesium level leads to a low intracellular potassium level related to the effect on the kidney causing an inability to conserve potassium in the tubules. As a result, hypokalemia may not be successfully treated until the magnesium level returns to normal range. The concurrent presence of hypokalemia with hypomagnesemia elevates the risk of cardiac dysrhythmias. Frequently, patients with hypomag-nesemia also experience hypocalcemia, particularly in moderate to severe stages of hypomagnesemia. Hypocalcemia occurs with hypo-magnesemia because a magnesium deficiency leads to decreased production of vitamin D, vitamin D resistance, and decreased intes-tinal calcium absorption. Neuromuscular excitability may occur with hypomagnesemia because a low magnesium level increases acetylcholine release from the nerve fibers. Neuromuscular excitability may be seen as weakness, tremors, hyperreflexia and seizures. Seizures are exhibited at low serum magnesium levels, especially in children.

Hypomagnesemia Assessment

- Electrolyte disturbances
  - Hypokalemia
  - Hypocalcemia
- Weakness
- Confusion/agitation
- Tetany/seizures

Hypomagnesemia Interpretation Criteria

The dysrhythmias that result from reduced serum magnesium levels are to some extent due to a reduction in the activity of ATPase at the sodium–potassium pump, plus reduced DNA and RNA metabolism. Hypomagnesemia may increase the incidence of cardiac dysrhythmias by reducing the intracellular potassium, leading to the development of reentrant circuits causing atrial tachycardias, atrial fibrillation, torsade de pointes, and ventricular fibrillation. Hypomagnesemia has been linked to an increased risk for ventricular dysrhythmias 5 to 12 days after a myocardial infarction. Hypomagnesemia in the presence of digoxin toxicity increases the risk of dysrhythmias (Fig. 8-3).

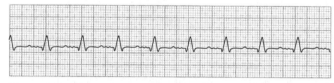

Figure 8-3   Hypomagnesemia.

Hypomagnesemia Interpretation Criteria

1. Rhythm: regular
2. Rate: 60–100 bpm
3. P wave: flattened P waves
4. PRI: greater than 0.20 sec
5. QRS I: slightly greater than 0.12 sec with decreased height of QRS wave
6. Other: discernible U waves and flat T waves with prolonged QT interval

Hypomagnesemia Care Measures

Assessing the patient for signs and symptoms of hypomagnesemia and drawing serum magnesium levels is the necessary first step in caring for patients with this electrolyte disturbance. Both the hypocalcemia and the hypokalemia associated with hypomagnesemia are treated by replacing magnesium prior to, or concurrently with, calcium and potassium supplements. Magnesium may be replaced either orally or parenterally dependent on serum levels and physical status. Dietary sources of magnesium include foods such as whole-grain cereals, nuts, seafood, and soybeans. Intracellular levels of magnesium may take up to 48 hours for complete replacement. Magnesium sulfate is administered intravenously at a dosage of 2 g over 1 to 2 minutes for torsades de pointes. For tonic-clonic seizures, magnesium sulfate is administered at a dosage of 2 g over 10 minutes. Other than for torsades de pointes or tonic-clonic seizures, magnesium sulfate parenterally is usually administered diluted at 1 to 4 g/hr. Prophylactic and early treatment of magnesium replacement is given for several days after a myocardial infarction. Oral dosing with a magnesium supplement is considered necessary when the cause of the hypomagnesemia is unable to be treated.

Hypomagnesemia Care Measures

* Assess impact of the rhythm on the patient's clinical signs and symptoms
* Administer magnesium replacement orally or parenterally
* Administer calcium gluconate and potassium chloride

Hypermagnesemia

Hypermagnesemia is more rarely observed than hypomagnesemia. Hypermagnesemia is described as a serum magnesium level of greater than 2.4 mg/dL or 2.0 mEq/L. An elevated serum magnesium level works effectively to block the movement of calcium extracellularly and intracellularly, leading to a prolongation of the PRI, increased QRS I width, and increased QT interval, which can eventually evolve into third-degree heart block and asystole.

Hypermagnesemia Causes

A common cause of hypermagnesemia is the administration of magnesium-based laxatives/antacids and supplements, particularly in patients with diminished renal function. Oliguric or anuric stages of acute or chronic renal failure cause decreased renal excretion of magnesium.

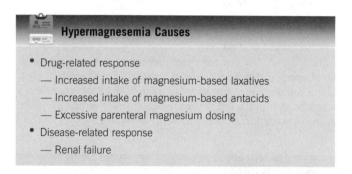

Hypermagnesemia Causes

- Drug-related response
  — Increased intake of magnesium-based laxatives
  — Increased intake of magnesium-based antacids
  — Excessive parenteral magnesium dosing
- Disease-related response
  — Renal failure

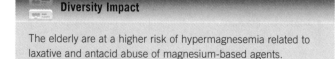

Diversity Impact

The elderly are at a higher risk of hypermagnesemia related to laxative and antacid abuse of magnesium-based agents.

Hypermagnesemia Assessment

The most common symptoms of hypermagnesemia are due to neuromuscular transmission blockage resulting in weakness and lack of deep tendon reflexes that may progress to paralysis of skeletal and respiratory muscles. As the magnesium levels rise, the neuromuscular end-plates inhibit the release of acetylcholine, leading to a loss of neuromuscular function. Hypermagnesemia produces a negative inotropic effect causing hypotension due to a decrease in strength of the cardiac contractions. At 5.0 to 6.0 mEq/L, vasodilation and hypotension occur due to vascular smooth muscle relaxation. Symptoms are more likely to be exhibited when the serum levels rise quickly.

Hypermagnesemia Assessment

Mild	Moderate	Severe
4.0–6.0 mEq/L, 4.8–7.2 mg/dL or 2–3 mmol/L	6.0–10.0 mEq/L, 7.2–12 mg/dL, or 3–5 mmol/L	> 10 mEq/L, 12 mg/dL, or 5 mmol/L
Nausea	Vasodilatation	Asystole
Lack of deep tendon reflexes	Hypocalcemia	Respiratory failure
Weakness	Bradycardia	Coma
	Hypotension	

Hypermagnesemia Interpretation Criteria

In hypermagnesemia, the cell membrane is stabilized, which lessens the automaticity and after depolarizations slowing down the AV and ventricular conduction. As the level of magnesium rises within the bloodstream, the PRI becomes greater than 0.20 seconds, producing AV conduction delays that could extend to a third-degree heart block and eventually asystole. Even at levels of 4.5 mEq/L, the sinus node may be depressed, causing the atria to take over the automaticity function of the heart in the form of atrial fibrillation. At levels of higher than 15 mEq/L, heart blocks and the risk for asystole become high (Fig. 8-4).

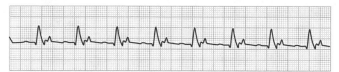

Figure 8-4   Hypermagnesemia.

Hypermagnesemia Interpretation Criteria

1. Rhythm: regular
2. Rate: 60–100 bpm
3. P wave: upright, uniform, and flattened
4. PRI: greater than 0.20 sec
5. QRS I: greater than 0.12 sec
6. Other: tented T wave

Hypermagnesemia Care Measures

After assessing the patient for the signs and symptoms associated with hypermagnesemia and drawing serum magnesium levels, the next step is to decrease magnesium intake by limiting intake from diet and medications. At times, intravenous saline infusions may be given to diurese and promote the excretion of magnesium in patients with normal cardiac and renal function. Intravenous saline infusions have a down side in that they can cause hypocalcemia, which elevates the serum magnesium even higher. The administration of calcium gluconate intravenously decreases the risk for lethal dysrhythmias. Careful monitoring of all serum electrolytes during hypermagnesemia treatment is essential. Hemodialysis or peritoneal dialysis may be used for severely elevated magnesium levels and patients in renal failure. Because magnesium acts naturally within the heart as a calcium channel blocker, calcium gluconate may be administered as an antagonist to counteract the effect of magnesium at the cell membrane, particularly if the patient has dysrhythmias, hypotension, or respiratory paralysis.

Hypermagnesemia Care Measures

- Assess impact of the rhythm on the patient's clinical signs and symptoms.
- Decrease dietary intake of magnesium.
- Eliminate magnesium-based laxatives/antacids from regimen.
- Administer calcium intravenously.
- Perform hemodialysis.

CALCIUM

Normal serum calcium levels range from 8.7 to 10.4 mg/dL. Ionized serum calcium levels range from 4.5 to 5.1 mg/dL and are more reflective of the actual amount of free calcium available for heart function than the total serum calcium level. Most calcium is found within the bone (99%), with the remaining 1% found attached to anions (10%), bound to proteins (40%), or in an ionized state (50%). Total serum calcium levels reflect calcium that is bound to protein. In cases of hypoalbuminemia, the total serum calcium level needs to be adjusted through the use of a mathematical calculation to reflect the amounts of calcium bound to protein. Consequently, ionized calcium levels may be obtained to more easily evaluate the amount of calcium available for cardiac functioning. See the calculation on the next page when ionized calcium levels are unavailable. The corrected calcium level range is 9.0 to 10.6 mg/dL.

Mathematical Calculation Determining Effect of Albumin on Total Serum Calcium Levels

Formula

Total serum calcium level in mg/dL + 0.8 (4.4 – Serum albumin level g/dL) = Corrected calcium level

Example of patient with hypoalbuminemia yet with normal serum calcium level

Albumin level 3.2 g/dL, total serum calcium level 8.1 mg/dL

$$8.1 \text{ mg/dL} + 0.8 (4.4 - 3.2 \text{ g/dL}) = 9.06 \text{ mg/dL}$$

Calcium level would not be treated for this patient.

Example of patient with hypoalbuminemia who *is* hypercalcemic

Albumin level 2.9 g/dL, total serum calcium level 10.1 mg/dL

$$10.1 \text{ mg/dL} + 0.8 (4.4 - 2.9 \text{ g/dL}) = 12.18 \text{ mg/dL}$$

Calcium level would be treated for this patient.

(Normal range of serum albumin: 3.5–5.0 mg/dL)

Calcium levels are regulated by three hormones: calcitriol, calcitonin, and parathyroid hormones. Calcium is necessary in the heart for both electrical and mechanical functioning in a multitude of ways. When the cell depolarizes, calcium levels rise in the sarcoplasmic reticulum, and calcium attaches onto troponin, which triggers the sliding action of the actin and myosin filaments across each other, resulting in muscle contraction. Calcium moves into the cardiac muscle cell after depolarization simultaneously with potassium movement out of the cell, creating a plateau phase and lengthening the action potential, which spurs repolarization. An inverse relationship exists between the calcium level and the QT interval. As the calcium level decreases, the QT interval becomes prolonged; and as the calcium level increases, the QT interval becomes shortened.

Hypocalcemia

Hypocalcemia is described as a total serum calcium level of less than 8.7 mg/dL or an ionized calcium level of less than 4.5 mg/dL. Lower serum calcium levels alter the action potential duration, particularly in phase 2, which leads to a prolongation of the QT interval.

Hypocalcemia Causes

Hypocalcemia may occur for a multitude of reasons ranging from inadequate intake, to malabsorption, to increased loss of calcium via renal or intestinal excretion, to other electrolyte imbalances or to disease states. Inadequate dietary intake of calcium and/or vitamin D can lead to hypocalcemia. Hypocalcemia may evolve as an adverse effect from pharmacotherapy. Low magnesium levels prevent the activation of the calcium feedback loop, resulting in higher excretion rates via the kidney and intestinal tract. Hypomagnesemia may be found in alcoholism or malabsorption syndromes. Higher serum levels of phosphate increase the binding of calcium to phosphate, precipitating salt deposition in the tissues and decreasing serum calcium levels. High phosphate levels may be found in patients with frequent Fleet enemas and neonates receiving cow's milk or high phosphate formula. In alkalotic states, protein has an increased affinity and binding to calcium, resulting in a decreased serum ionized calcium level. Citrate is a preservative in packed red blood cells that attaches to extracellular calcium, depleting the ionized calcium reserves within the bloodstream. The parathyroid gland has the primary responsibility for controlling serum calcium levels. When the parathyroid gland fails to secrete parathyroid hormone, calcium uptake by the intestines, reabsorption by the kidneys, and bone mobilization fail to function, resulting in hypocalcemia. Hypoparathyroidism may occur congenitally or as a complication after a thyroidectomy. In renal failure, low serum calcium levels are seen related to inability of the kidneys to convert vitamin D to its active metabolites and hyperphosphatemia due to reduced glomerular filtration rates. In pancreatitis, hypocalcemia may occur due to hypoalbuminemia, malnutrition, and calcium salt deposition in the retroperitoneum.

Hypocalcemia Causes

- Drug-related response
  - Biphosphonates
  - Calcitonin
  - Selective serotonin uptake inhibitors
  - Proton pump inhibitors
  - Chelating agents (CDC, 2006)
- Disease-related response
  - Parathyroid deficiency
  - Renal failure
  - Pancreatitis
  - Hypoalbuminemia
  - Acid–base/electrolyte imbalances
    - Alkalosis
    - Hypomagnesemia
    - Hyperphosphatemia

Diversity Impact

A very high incidence of hypocalcemia is found in premature infants with gestational ages of less than 32 weeks, asphyxia at birth, and mothers with diabetes mellitus.

(Singhal, 2006)

Hypocalcemia Assessment

Symptoms typically occur when ionized calcium levels are less than 2.5 mg/dL. Chronic hypocalcemia may be asymptomatic, while acute hypocalcemia usually exhibits neuromuscular irritability. The first symptoms to arise are paresthesias in the face and extremities followed by positive Chvostek and Trousseau signs, which may eventually result in tetany and seizures as the level continues to drop (see Figures 8-5 and 8-6). Hypocalcemia leads to decreased cardiac contractility related to decreased amounts of calcium moving across the actin and myosin filaments for contraction to occur. Heart failure can result from the decreased myocardial contractility.

Hypocalcemia Assessment

- Asymptomatic
- Paresthesias
- Positive Chvostek and Trousseau signs
- Tetany/seizures
- Heart failure

Chvostek and Trousseau Signs

Chvostek Sign
Tapping of cranial nerve VII (facial nerve) near the ear elicits spasm of the cheek muscle, lip, nose, and eye

Figure 8-5   Chvostek sign.

Trousseau Sign
Inflation of the blood pressure cuff to 20 mm Hg above the patient's blood pressure for 2 minutes elicits carpal spasm

Figure 8-6   Trousseau sign.

Hypocalcemia Interpretation Criteria

Hypocalcemia prolongs the action potential duration time of phase 2 of the cardiac cycle creating the classic ECG change associated with hypocalcemia of a prolonged QT interval of greater than 0.44 seconds with a flat, long ST segment. A prolonged QT interval increases the risk for patients to develop torsades de pointes (Fig. 8-7).

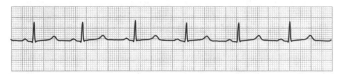

Figure 8-7   Hypocalcemia.

Hypocalcemia Interpretation Criteria

1. Rhythm: regular
2. Rate: 60–100 bpm
3. P wave: upright, uniform, and round
4. PRI: 0.12–0.20 sec
5. QRS I: less than 0.12 sec
6. Other: flat, long ST segment with prolonged QT interval greater than 0.44 sec

Hypocalcemia Care Measures

The first step is to assess for the associated signs and symptoms of hypocalcemia and obtain total serum calcium and/or ionized serum calcium levels. Simultaneously, other laboratory values may need to be assessed, as calcium tends not to operate in a vacuum or by itself; therefore, assess magnesium, potassium, phosphorus, albumin, vitamin D, and serum pH. Treatment of asymptomatic patients is controversial and the main thrust felt to be needed is to treat the cause of the hypocalcemia. Magnesium, potassium, and pH levels need to be treated at the same time as the calcium. For example, an untreated magnesium level will make the patient unable to respond appropriately to calcium treatment. Dietary sources of calcium include dairy (milk, yogurt, cheese) as well as salmon, baked beans, and oranges. When the hypocalcemia results due to renal failure or hypoparathyroidism, administration of vitamin D and oral calcium may be necessary for the remaining part of the patient's life. Phosphate binders may be given to lower serum phosphate levels. For acute hypocalcemia with symptoms, intravenous calcium administration may be needed to raise the level. Calcium gluconate is preferred intravenous therapy over calcium chloride, because calcium chloride has a higher risk of extravasation.

Hypocalcemia Care Measures

- Assess impact of the rhythm on the patient's clinical signs and symptoms.
- Evaluate other laboratory tests: magnesium, phosphate, albumin, potassium, and serum pH.
- Encourage intake of foods high in calcium
- Administer magnesium concurrently with calcium replacement.
- Administer calcium supplements orally or intravenously.
- Administer vitamin D.

Hypercalcemia

Hypercalcemia is described as a total serum calcium level of greater than 10.4 mg/dL or an ionized serum calcium level of greater than 5.1 mg/dL. Elevated levels of calcium decreases the plateau phase of the action potential, resulting in a shorter ST segment, which creates a depressant effect on the heart. Initially, higher serum calcium levels may increase contractility of the myocardium, but when the level reaches higher than 16 mg/dL, the opposite effect may occur.

Hypercalcemia Causes

The two main causes of hypercalcemia are hyperparathyroidism and cancer. In hyperparathyroidism, parathyroid hormone production is increased, leading to increased calcitriol secretion, causing increased calcium absorption by the intestine; and the parathyroid hormone decreases the excretion of calcium by the distal tubules of the kidney. Three main types of cancer that may lead to the release of calcium from the bones are multiple myeloma, lung cancer, and breast cancer. Hypercalcemia may also occur from metastasis of the cancer to the bone. When patients are immobile and unable to bear weight by standing or sitting, bones start to release calcium into the extracellular spaces, yielding hypercalcemia. As is expected, an increase in dietary calcium or intake of excessive amounts of calcium supplements or calcium-based antacids may increase the serum calcium level, causing hypercalcemia. Thiazide diuretics decrease the renal excretion of calcium. Granulomatous diseases such as tuberculosis and sarcoidosis increase calcitriol levels, leading to hypercalcemia. Calcitriol stimulates the absorption of calcium from the intestinal tract. In an acidotic state, protein and calcium have a decreased affinity for each other, resulting in an increased ionized calcium level. When phosphorus levels drop, more calcium is absorbed from the intestines.

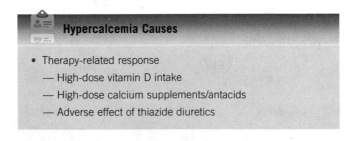

Hypercalcemia Causes

- Therapy-related response
  — High-dose vitamin D intake
  — High-dose calcium supplements/antacids
  — Adverse effect of thiazide diuretics

- Disease-related response
  — Immobility
  — Acid–base/electrolyte imbalance
    ▪ Acidosis
    ▪ Hypophosphatemia
  — Cancer
  — Hyperparathyroidism
  — Granulomatous diseases

Diversity Impact

Hyperparathyroidism has a higher incidence in women than men. Cancer and hyperparathyroidism incidence increases with age leading to higher risk with older individuals.

Hypercalcemia Assessment

Hypercalcemia is usually asymptomatic for mildly elevated serum calcium levels. Older patients may exhibit more symptoms of hypercalcemia than younger patients will. As serum calcium levels rise, cell membranes become less excitable. Nausea and vomiting are usually the first two symptoms to appear. The depressant effects of excess calcium leads to weakness, constipation, muscle aches, and decreased muscle tone. The weakness and joint aches are usually worse in the lower extremities. Abdominal and flank pain may reflect symptoms of renal lithiasis due to calcium-based stones in the renal tubules. Coma may occur with very high levels of calcium. A reflection of the clinical signs and symptoms has resulted in the development of a mnemonic to depict the main components— "stones, bones, abdominal moans, and psychic groans."

Hypercalcemia Lab Values

Mild	Moderate	Severe

Total Ca$^+$
  10.4–11.9 mg/dL
	Total Ca$^+$
	  12.0–13.9 mg/dL
		Total Ca$^+$
		  14–16 mg/dL

Ionized Ca$^+$
  5.6–8 mg/dL
	Ionized Ca$^+$
	  8.1–9.9 mg/dL
		Ionized Ca$^+$
		  10–12 mg/dL

Hypercalcemia Assessment

- Asymptomatic
- Nausea/vomiting/constipation
- Abdominal/flank pain
- Weakness/joint aches
- Lethargy/confusion/coma

Hypercalcemia Interpretation Criteria

The main ECG change seen in hypercalcemia is a short ST segment with the T wave originating immediately upon completion of the QRS complex. Elevated serum calcium levels shorten the plateau phase of the cardiac action potential, leading to a delay of the AV conduction and first-degree heart block. ECG changes from hypercalcemia are infrequently observed. Rarely, ST segment elevation occurs with hypercalcemia, and is often originally considered to be a myocardial infarction until coronary angiogram and troponin levels rule out the MI (Nishi et al., 2006). See Figure 8-8.

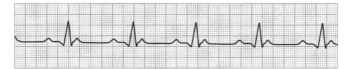

Figure 8-8 Hypercalcemia.

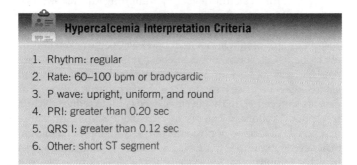

Hypercalcemia Interpretation Criteria

1. Rhythm: regular
2. Rate: 60–100 bpm or bradycardic
3. P wave: upright, uniform, and round
4. PRI: greater than 0.20 sec
5. QRS I: greater than 0.12 sec
6. Other: short ST segment

Hypercalcemia Care Measures

Symptoms are less reliable as an indicator of the level of hypercalcemia. But, that being said, the first step is still to assess for the effects of the rhythm on the patient as well as obtain the serum electrolyte level. Hypercalcemia exhibits itself in other systems, mostly the gastrointestinal and musculoskeletal areas. Obviously, one of the first measures is to discontinue the intake of calcium-rich foods/supplements/antacids. Mobilization of the patient safely will drive the calcium back into the bone. When the serum calcium level reaches 14 mg/dL or is symptomatic at levels higher than 12 mg/dL, treatment is begun to lower the level. One method is the administration of intravenous normal saline at larger volumes, usually about 200 mL/hr, to flush the calcium out of the body via the urine. The sodium in a normal saline IV solution decreases the reabsorption of calcium by the kidney. At times, the administration of furosemide is needed to "jump start" the kidneys and facilitate the removal of the excess fluid. Treatment of hypercalcemia with furosemide is controversial, as it could promote the release of calcium from the bone; yet furosemide is definitely needed in patients with heart failure. Thiazide diuretics are **not** used due to their blockage of calcium excretion by the kidneys. Bisphosphonates decrease serum calcium levels by inhibiting the breakdown of bones. Persistent elevations of calcium may be treated with corticosteroids and calcitonin. Corticosteroids reduce calcium absorption from the intestine and promote calcium excretion by the kidneys. Calcitonin suppresses bone resorption and promotes renal excretion of calcium. Surgery and removal of the parathyroid glands may be necessary to treat hyperparathyroidism. For patients with cancer, mithramycin may be given to reduce calcium resorption by bones. Patients in renal failure or heart failure may need hemodialysis or peritoneal dialysis with low or no calcium dialysate solutions to lower their calcium levels. Chelating agents may be administered for extremely high calcium levels, but there are risks associated with use of these agents.

Hypercalcemia Care Measures

- Assess impact of the rhythm on the patient's clinical signs and symptoms.
- Decrease intake of calcium-rich foods.
- Mobilize safely when able.
- Administer intravenous saline hydration.
- Administer furosemide (controversial).
- Administer bisphosphonates.
- Administer mithramycin.
- Perform hemodialysis/peritoneal dialysis.
- Administer chelating agents.

REFERENCES

Al-Momen A, El-Mogy I. Intragastric balloon for obesity: a retrospective evaluation of tolerance and efficacy. *Obes Surg*. 2005;15:101–105.

Centers for Disease Control and Prevention (CDC). Deaths associated with hypocalcemia from chelation therapy—Texas, Pennsylvania, and Oregon, 2003–2005. *MMWR Weekly*. 2006;55;204–207. Retrieved on November 19, 2008 from http://www.cdc.gov/mmwr/preview/mmwrhtm/mm5508a3.htm.

Cheng CJ, Lin CS, Chang LW. Perplexing hyperkalemia. *Nephrol Dial Transplant*. 2006;21:3320–3323.

Fang J, Madhavan S, Alderman MH. Dietary potassium intake and stroke mortality. *Stroke*. 2000;31:1532–1537

Garth D. Hypokalemia. 2007. Retrieved on November 15, 2008 from http://www.emedicine.com/emerg/topic273.htm.

Hollander-Rodriguez JC, Calvert JF. Hyperkalemia. *Am Fam Physician*. 2006;73:283–290.

Lederer E. Hyperkalemia. 2009. Retrieved on June 5, 2009 from http://www.emedicine.com/med/article/240903-overview.

Nishi S, Barbagelata N, Atar S, Birnbaum Y, Tuero F. Hypercalcemia-induced ST segment elevation mimicking acute myocardial infarction. *J Electrocardiol*. 2006;39:298–300.

Novello NP, Blumstein HA. Hypermagnesemia. 2007. Retrieved on November 20, 2008 from http://www.emedicine.com/emerg/topic262.htm.

Singhal A. Hypocalcemia. 2006. Retrieved on October 16, 2008 from http://www.emedicine.com/ped/topic1111.htm.

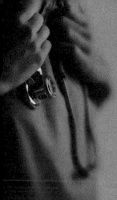

Chapter 9
MYOCARDIAL INFARCTION

A myocardial infarction (MI) is an insufficient oxygen supply compared to oxygen demand in the cardiac tissue, resulting in cell necrosis. The left ventricle is considered the "powerhouse" of the heart, having the thickest myocardial wall and using the most blood supply from the coronary arteries. Smaller branches of the coronary arteries supply the other three chambers of the heart. Occlusion of coronary arteries will most typically affect the left ventricle. As a result, the electrical conduction pathways are evaluated in the left ventricle to determine the location of an infarction. The infarcted area of the heart does not depolarize or contract, leading to impaired left ventricular function. Areas of ischemia and injury that surround the infarcted tissue are hypoxic and can cause dangerous ventricular ectopy and rhythms.

More than 50% of the deaths from a myocardial infarction occur before the patient reaches the hospital. The mortality rate within the hospital from a myocardial infarction appears to be about 10%, with another 10% of the deaths occurring within the first year after an infarct. For a long period of time, myocardial infarctions have been a major health issue in the industrialized world, but the World Heart Federation projects a sharp increase in developing countries, particularly Latin America, Asia, and Eastern Europe.

MYOCARDIAL INFARCTION CAUSES

The main reasons for the inequality in oxygen supply and demand are from atherosclerosis, thrombus, embolism, vasospasm in the coronary arteries, or decreased ventricular filling time. The definition of myocardial infarctions has recently been redefined to reflect scientific and societal changes in the field. The new definition addresses the cause of the infarct as either spontaneous or procedure-related, amount of cell necrosis or infarct size, and the timing of patient observation to the time of myocardial necrosis as either acute, healing, or healed (Thygesen et al., 2007). The acute phase of a myocardial infarction refers to the time period from 6 hours to 7 days. The healing phase time period is from 7 to 28 days, while the healed phase exists after 29 days. Each of the phases correlates to the pathophysiologic state occurring within each time period and may be estimated through a form of echocardiography (RT3DE).

Categories of myocardial infarction are classified into five types: (1) spontaneous, related to ischemia from plaque erosion and/or fissuring, rupturing, or dissection; (2) ischemia from oxygen supply and demand inequality (anemia, embolism, dysrhythmias, hypertension/hypotension, or coronary artery spasm); (3) sudden cardiac death; (4) procedural, related to percutaneous coronary interventions or stent thrombosis; or (5) surgical, related to coronary artery bypass graft (Thygesen et al., 2007). Ninety percent of myocardial infarctions are due to atheromatous plaque formation narrowing the blood vessels followed by a plaque rupture leading to platelet aggregation, clot formation, accumulation of fibrin, and vasospasm resulting in complete occlusion of the blood vessel. Atheromatous plaques grow over time as part of an inflammatory process and are composed of a fibromuscular cap with an underlying soft lipid core. Over years, enzymes erode and thin the fibromuscular cap, creating fissures, ulcerations, and structural instability, particularly near the vessel wall. When the endothelial wall is disrupted, platelet aggregation can occur, creating a thrombus that may occlude the coronary vessel, causing a myocardial infarction. Other causes of a myocardial infarction resulting from inequality of oxygen supply and demand and inadequate blood flow to the cardiac muscle include disorders such as chest trauma from motor vehicle crashes, emboli, and gastrointestinal bleeding. Massive gastrointestinal bleeding and hypoxia from various pulmonary disorders decrease the oxygen supply to the heart by either decreasing the oxygen-carrying capacity through decreased hemoglobin levels from bleeding or through decreased ability to either extract or attain oxygen in the pulmonary system.

Risk factors for a myocardial infarction are categorized as non-modifiable and modifiable. Non-modifiable risk factors are ones that are unable to be changed within an individual such as age, gender, ethnicity, and family history. Men have a higher predilection for an infarct between the ages of 40 and 70 years than women do. In the United States, 50% of myocardial infarctions occur in individuals less than 65 years of age. Under the age of 45, risk factors include cocaine use, type I diabetes mellitus, hypercholesteremia, and family history for early coronary artery disease. Family screening needs to be focused on myocardial infarctions in men under the age of 45 and women under the age of 55. Higher incidences of myocardial infarction have been found in Caucasian men and Asian Indians, with lower incidences seen in Japanese and French populations. Modifiable risk factors are ones under a patient's control to change such as smoking, alcohol intake, high cholesterol levels, obesity, sedentary lifestyle, cocaine use, diabetes, and hypertension.

Diversity Impact

Typically, myocardial infarction occurs after the age of 45, with a higher incidence in men versus women until the age of 70. An increased incidence of myocardial infarctions is found in Caucasian men and Asian Indians, with lower incidences seen in French and Japanese individuals.

Myocardial Infarction Causes

- Disease-related response
  - Atherosclerotic plaque fissure, rupture, or dissection
  - Decreased oxygen supply or increased oxygen demand
    - Anemia
    - Embolism
    - Dysrhythmias
    - Hypertension/hypotension
    - Coronary artery spasm
  - Sudden cardiac death
  - Procedural
    - Percutaneous coronary intervention
    - Stent thrombosis
    - Thrombolytic therapy
  - Coronary artery bypass graft

MYOCARDIAL INFARCTION DIAGNOSIS

Similar to the dysrhythmia discussion, interpretation of ECG changes in possible MI patients needs to be completed holistically. The gold standard for diagnosing a myocardial infarction are the history and physical assessment, evaluation of troponin levels, and the ECG. Evaluation of ECG changes can be a helpful tool when diagnosing a myocardial infarction, but needs to be used in conjunction with a history and physical assessment and evaluation of serum cardiac markers.

History and Physical Assessment

The classic symptom of a myocardial infarction is chest pain. Unfortunately, chest pain may be associated with a wide variety of health issues that may be life-threatening or of a minor consequence. Anginal chest pain sometimes may be differentiated from myocardial infarction pain through assessment of duration of chest pain, precipitating factors of the chest pain, dysrhythmias accompanying the chest pain, and presence of associated signs and symptoms. The main difference between anginal and infarction chest pain is that myocardial infarction pain lasts longer than 20 minutes and is unrelieved by rest. Noncardiac causes of chest pain are numerous, such as inflammation of the pericardial sac (pericarditis), chest trauma (myocardial contusion), overuse of the chest muscles (muscle strain), or build up of air, fluid, or blood in the pleural cavity (hemo/pneumo/tension pneumothorax).Until a myocardial infarction is ruled out, the complaint of chest pain is considered to be of a cardiac origin.

Only about 10% of patients who present in the emergency department with chest pain have had a myocardial infarction. A decrease in oxygen supply or increase in oxygen demand in the cardiac tissue can cause lactic acid to be produced in the tissue and pain to be felt by the patient. Myocardial infarction chest pain usually lasts longer than 20 to 30 minutes, may be located in the substernal chest area, jaw, neck, upper back, or radiate down the left arm. The chest pain can be described as sharp, stabbing, "an elephant sitting on my chest," a heaviness, dull ache, or indigestion. Patients with diabetes mellitus, paralysis, or heart transplants may not experience any chest pain. Other populations who may experience atypical chest pain or no chest pain at all are women and the elderly. About 10% of all myocardial infarctions are "silent," meaning that the patient presents without any chest pain. Women may present with fatigue, sleep disturbances, shortness of breath, indigestion, and anxiety. Elderly patients may present with profound weakness, confusion, and fatigue. Associated symptoms in a myocardial infarction are diaphoresis, shortness of breath, nausea, vomiting, and changes in vital signs. Anxiety may evolve with a sense of impending doom as the body senses an issue. Denial of chest pain is a common occurrence. Frequently, patients may refer to their chest pain as "indigestion" and feel that the pain will subside shortly, resulting in a delay in seeking treatment (Table 9-1).

Diversity Impact

Women may present with fatigue, sleep disturbances, and shortness of breath. The elderly may present with profound weakness, confusion, or fatigue.

History and Physical Assessment

- Chest pain
- Diaphoresis
- Shortness of breath
- Nausea and vomiting
- Vital sign changes

Table 9-1   Differentiation of Anginal versus Myocardial Infarction Chest Pain

Criteria	Angina Pectoris	Myocardial Infarction
Duration of Chest Pain	Less than 20 min	Greater than 20 min
Precipitating Factors	Usually precipitated by stress and exercise, relieved by rest	Not precipitated by stress & exercise; unrelieved by rest
Accompanied by Dysrhythmias	No dysrhythmias	Dysrhythmias noted
Associated Signs & Symptoms	Usually none	Usually present
Response to Nitroglycerin	Pain responds to less than three nitroglycerin tablets	Not relieved by nitroglycerin

Serum Cardiac Markers

When cardiac cells die, the cell's contents, including biochemical markers, are released into the bloodstream. The biochemical markers released are creatine kinase, particularly the MB; troponin I, troponin T, and myoglobin. Two newer forms of cardiac markers are ischemia-modified albumin (IMA) and heart–fatty acid-binding protein, which are released by cardiac tissue within minutes of ischemia. Research is still pending on the ability of these biochemical markers to predict serious cardiac outcomes (Charpentier, 2009). All of these cardiac markers can be informative to document the extent of cellular death and to calculate the approximate timing of the infarct. Each cardiac marker has a detection point, peak, and duration of time of elevation within the serum. Detection, peak, and duration of elevation for each of the markers can provide information on timing of the beginning of the infarct. Review of detection, peak, and duration levels of cardiac markers is especially helpful in determining treatment for individuals with "silent" MI's or individuals who deny the possibility of an MI and delay seeking treatment. Serial cardiac markers need to be obtained to rule in/out a myocardial infarction. Do not rely on a single blood sample! Myoglobin increases when either skeletal or cardiac cell damage occurs, and is the first of the current serum markers to become elevated after an infarction. The creatine kinase MB has a higher specificity, as it predominantly increases after myocardial necrosis whereas myoglobin may increase with both skeletal muscle damage and cardiac muscle damage. Calculation of the CK-MB mass index requires serum lab draws at 2, 4, and 6 hours to analyze the slope of change over time and determine the probability of a myocardial infarction. Troponin I and troponin T are cardiac specific and elevate with both myocardial infarction and myocardial injury, improving their diagnostic abilities. Troponin levels need to be drawn 6 hours apart. Since the serum markers for myocardial necrosis require a minimum of 20 minutes to determine their levels in the laboratory, initial diagnosis and treatment is based on clinical assessment and ECG interpretation. Rapid troponin T levels are now able to be drawn and evaluated right at the bedside, increasing its usefulness for diagnosing an MI quickly. Troponin T and troponin I are now considered to be the gold standard for diagnosing an MI related to their high cardiac tissue specificity and high sensitivity. Unfortunately, troponin T can also be elevated in renal failure and other muscular disorders. For early diagnosis, the CK-MB mass or myoglobin levels may be added to the cardiac panel that already includes troponin levels. Two other laboratory tests that may support the diagnosis of an infarction are an elevated white blood cell count and an elevated serum C-reactive protein level. Definitive diagnosis of a myocardial infarction is based on rise and fall of troponins and CK-MB, plus ischemia symptoms, pathologic Q waves, ST segment elevation, or stenosis/ obstruction found in a coronary angiogram. ECG changes of ST segment elevation/depression and T-wave inversion are not sufficient on their own to definitively diagnose a myocardial infarction. Serum cardiac markers are summarized in Table 9-2.

Table 9-2   Serum Cardiac Markers

Cardiac Marker	Level Indicating MI	Detection (hr)	Peak (hr)	Duration of Elevation
Troponin I	>0.4 ng/mL = MI >0.06 ng/mL = high risk of ACS or nonischemic myocardial damage <0.06 ng/mL on two specimens >6 hr apart = unstable angina	4–12	12–24	5–7 days
Troponin T	>0.1 ng/mL = MI <0.03 ng/mL = on two specimens >6 hr apart = unstable angina	4–12	12–48	5–15 days
CK-MB mass	>8.0 ng/mL Slope of log CK-MB/hr >0.03	3–6	12–24	1–2 days
Myoglobin	>90 ng/mL; doubling of value in 1–2 hr = MI	1–4	6–7	24 hr

MYOCARDIAL INFARCTION ECG INTERPRETATION CRITERIA

An ECG needs to be obtained as early as possible from the onset of chest pain or determination of the possibility of a myocardial infarction. ECGs may be or may not be diagnostic of a myocardial infarction due to variations between individual's anatomic location, coronary vessels, and heart structure. Serial ECGs and comparison of current ECG to previously obtained ones can be more informative and diagnostic at times. When assessing a 12-lead ECG for a myocardial infarction, the first action is to stay consistent in the approach by applying the five-step approach of interpreting the rhythm, rate, P waves, PRI, and QRS I. For a myocardial infarction, three additional steps are added: (1) determining the presence of T-wave inversion and ST segment depression, (2) assessing for ST segment elevation, and (3) evaluating the existence of a pathological Q wave. Evaluation of a 12-lead ECG for a myocardial infarction requires assessing for three levels of myocardial damage and determining the location of the infarcted area. Be aware that despite a normal ECG, the patient could still have had an MI. Four issues may confound the diagnosis of a myocardial infarction via an ECG including bundle branch block, Wolff–Parkinson–White syndrome, left ventricular hypertrophy, and postcoronary artery bypass graft surgery.

Stages of Myocardial Damage

Coronary blood vessel occlusion may cause three levels of damage, from ischemia to injury to infarction. Typically, at the time of the acute stages of infarction, three zones of damage occur distal to the occluded artery. The zone of infarction is the central area of necrotic or dead tissue, which is surrounded initially by a zone of injury, and then an outer layer called the zone of ischemia (Fig. 9-1). Myocardial wall damage was previously classified by the number of layers of damage to the wall: epicardium, myocardium, and endocardium. A subendocardial infarction extended only through the endocardium while a transmural myocardial infarction extended through all three layers of the myocardium. Currently, myocardial infarctions are categorized by the location of the damaged tissue and/or the presence or absence of Q waves or ST segment elevation. Yet movement to use the new classification system listed under "Myocardial Infarction Causes" earlier in the chapter can soon be expected to be within use in clinical arenas.

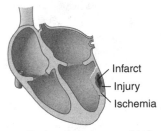

Figure 9-1   Zones of ischemia, injury, and infarction.

Ischemia

The first stage of myocardial damage evolves as oxygen supply becomes insufficient for the demand. The oxygen deprivation in the cardiac tissue creates classic ECG changes, including ST segment depression and changes in the T wave, initially peaking of the T wave and progressing to symmetrical T-wave inversion. The ST segment is from the end of the S wave to the beginning of the T wave and represents early repolarization of the ventricles. ST segment depression is considered indicative of ischemia when the ST segment is greater than 1 mm below the isoelectric line at 0.04 seconds to the right of the J point and is present in two or more contiguous leads. "J point" is the term for the location on the ECG where the QRS complex and ST segment meet. Contiguous leads are leads that view the same area of the heart electrically or chest leads in numeric consecutive order such as II, III, aVF; I, aVL; or V_1, V_2, V_3, V_4, V_5, V_6 (Table 9-3). ST segment depression may occur with or without

T-wave inversion. ST segment depression may be present with partial- or full-thickness myocardial wall ischemia.

Table 9-3   Contiguous Leads

- II, III, aVF
- I, aVL
- V_1, V_2, V_3, V_4, V_5, V_6

T-wave inversion occurs related to a leaking of potassium out of the ischemic cells, which delays repolarization. In the early stages of a myocardial infarction, the T wave may become tall and tented with a height of greater than 6 mm in limb leads and 12 mm in precordial leads. A rule of thumb is to assess the height of the T wave and the R wave. An abnormally high T wave is one that is greater than two thirds the size of the accompanying R wave. T-wave inversion indicates full-thickness myocardial wall ischemia. T wave inversion is most easily observed in the chest leads (V_1–V_6) located the closest to the ventricles (Fig. 9-2). Inversion of the T wave starts about 1 to 2 hours after the vessel becomes occluded and may persist for 1 to 3 days depending on the amount of collateral blood flow. When treated by improving oxygen delivery and decreasing oxygen demand by cardiac tissues, ischemia may be reversible, with T waves returning to baseline status of a positively deflected wave above the isoelectric line. When ischemia is associated with an infarction, T-wave inversion may be seen for several months after the ischemic event before returning to baseline. Besides myocardial ischemia, T-wave inversion may be caused by electrolyte imbalances, inflammation of the pericardial sac, right ventricular hypertrophy, bundle branch block, shock, and subarachnoid hemorrhage. Because T-wave inversion may be observed with other disorders, the ECG change is indicative of ischemia when the clinical symptoms support the diagnosis. In addition, inverted T waves associated with these other causes create T waves that are asymmetrical with a gentle downslope and rapid upslope.

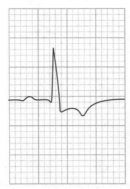

Figure 9-2   Myocardial ischemia ECG changes.

Ischemia may produce chest pain known as angina pectoris. Anginal pain may be experienced on and off for a period of many years or be a precursor to a myocardial infarction. Anginal pain from ischemia may be relieved by rest, oxygen, and nitroglycerin.

Injury

The second stage of myocardial damage occurs when the oxygen deprivation to the cardiac tissue occurs for a more prolonged time. For this stage, the classic ECG change is ST segment elevation in the leads consistent with the myocardial damaged areas. The ST segment elevation will be seen in at least two contiguous leads. Elevation of the ST segment of greater than 1 mm in limb leads and 2 mm in precordial leads at a point of 0.04 seconds to the right of the J point is indicative of myocardial injury. ST segment elevation may be seen for several days up to 2 weeks after an injury before returning to baseline. In the oxygen-deprived area of the myocardium, depolarization is incomplete and the injured area is more positive electrically than the surrounding uninjured area. ST segment elevation is one of the earliest signs indicating that a myocardial infarction has occurred (Fig. 9-3). ST segment elevation starts 20 to 40 minutes after the vessel becomes occluded and persists for about 1 to 3 days.

Besides myocardial injury, ST segment elevation may be caused by inflammation of the pericardium, hyperkalemia, pulmonary embolism, ventricular hypertrophy, and intracranial hemorrhage. Differentiation of the cause of ST segment elevation may be helped by observing the shape of the ST segment elevation and determining the presence of ST segment elevation in other leads. ST segment elevation from other causes than a myocardial infarction is usually present in all leads except for aVR and has a flatter or more concave shape. In a myocardial infarction, ST segment depression would be observed in the leads opposite the infarcted area. ST and T-wave abnormalities with normal cardiac serum markers are interpreted as being related to ischemia or injury, but not infarction.

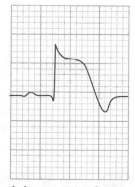

Figure 9-3   Myocardial injury ECG changes.

Injury may produce chest pain, which may be resolved if acted on quickly enough with treatments of fibrinolytic agents, percutaneous coronary interventions, or coronary artery bypass graft (CABG). When ST segment elevations are seen without a pathologic Q wave, the patient requires close monitoring and serial cardiac marker studies.

Infarction

The third stage of myocardial damage occurs when the cardiac tissue receives no oxygen for a prolonged time, resulting in necrosis. The necrotic damage is irreversible and in time will become scar tissue. For this stage, the classic ECG change is a pathologic Q wave, which may be seen hours to days after the initial insult. The change in the Q wave results from a lack of ventricular depolarization and indicates necrosis through the entire myocardial wall, commonly referred to as a Q-wave MI. Movement of the electrical activity away from the infarcted area creates a deep and negatively deflected Q wave. A pathologic Q wave is greater than or equal to 0.04 seconds wide and greater than one-third the height of the R wave in at least two contiguous leads over the infarcted area. (Fig. 9-4). Pathologic Q waves may be observed in 90% of ST segment elevated myocardial infarctions and 25% of non-ST segment elevated myocardial infarctions. The remaining patients are said to have a non-Q wave myocardial infarction. Presence or absence of Q waves was originally thought to be related to the number of layers of damage to the myocardial wall, but little correlation has been found between the presence of pathologic Q waves and transmural or subendocardial wall MIs. Non-Q wave infarctions will present with T-wave inversion and ST segment depression that lasts for longer than 48 hours. Non-Q wave MIs have been found to have lower initial mortality rates, but higher mortality rates overall when compared to Q wave MIs.

Diversity Impact

Significant Q waves in leads II, III, aVF, V_5, and V_6 may be normal in children, yet when seen in the remaining leads would be considered pathologic.

A second ECG change in infarction can be poor R-wave progression. In a normal R-wave progression, the R wave will become larger and the S wave will become smaller as the electrical activity moves from right to left across the chest leads

(V_1 to V_6). If the R wave does not become larger and the S wave does not become smaller in V_1–V_6, poor R-wave progression exists and may be helpful in diagnosing a variety of issues, from an anteroseptal MI, to a left bundle branch block, to chronic obstructive pulmonary disease.

Diagnosis of an MI may be considered when two or more contiguous leads have greater than 1 mm of ST segment elevation. Measure each small box vertically above the isoelectric line to the height of ST segment elevation. One small box equals 1 mm. Patients who develop Q waves may have them for several years or the rest of their life. Pathologic Q waves start to be seen about 2 to 24 hours after the vessel becomes occluded and may persist for the rest of the patient's life. In inferior wall myocardial infarctions, the Q wave may begin to decrease in size and width within 6 months.

The area of cell necrosis from artery blockage is surrounded by zones of injury and zones of ischemia. If the vessel is not reopened quickly, the zones of ischemia and injury may progress to a zone of infarction.

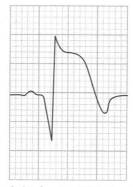

Figure 9-4 Myocardial infarction ECG changes.

Myocardial Infarction Location Sites

The location site of the myocardial infarction may impact treatment decisions and is predictive of possible complications. Five main locations are usually seen via a 12-lead ECG: anterior, inferior, lateral, septal, and posterior. Each location is associated with blockage of one or two coronary vessels. Combinations of infarctions in these five locations may be observed on ECG depending on the vessel involved, location within the vessel, and degree of occlusion such as anterolateral, anteroseptal, inferolateral, and posterolateral. (Fig. 9-5). Remember that each patient's anatomic location, vessels, and structure of the heart may vary; therefore the interpretation criteria discussed below are suggested as guidelines. The value of the ECG is tremendously improved when comparison to previous ECGs is possible.

Currently, newer methods using 15- or 18-lead ECGs may diagnose myocardial infarction sites and pinpoint the damaged areas with higher degrees of specificity. At more advanced levels of ECG interpretation, axis deviation and vector analysis become necessary components to understanding the ECG changes in 12-, 15-, and 18-lead ECGs. When evaluating the 12-lead ECG, both leads facing the infarcted area and leads opposite the infarcted area are assessed to determine the location site. Leads opposite the infarcted area are also called reciprocal leads. Each illustration depicting the location of infarction is shown with identification and placement of the leads facing the infarcted area and the leads opposite the infarcted area for easier understanding of the changes seen within an ECG for that particular location site. Lead aVR may not show changes in a myocardial infarction (Table 9-4).

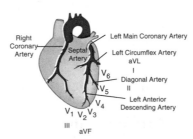

Figure 9-5   Vessel and lead involvement at myocardial infarction sites.

Table 9-4 Vessel and Lead Involvement at Myocardial Infarction Sites

Location	Vessel Occluded	Leads Facing Affected Area	Leads Opposite Affected Area
Anterior	Left anterior descending, diagonal branch	V_3, V_4	II, II, aVF
Inferior	Right coronary artery	II, III, aVF	I, aVL
Lateral	Left coronary artery	I, aVL, V_5, V_6	II, III, aVF
Septal	Left anterior descending, septal branch	V_1, V_2, V_3	V_7, V_8, V_9
Posterior	Posterior descending branch of right coronary artery or left circumflex artery	V_7, V_8, V_9	V_1, V_2, V_3, V_4

Anterior Wall Myocardial Infarction

An anterior wall myocardial infarction develops when the diagonal branch of the left anterior descending artery is occluded. Leads facing the infarcted area of an anterior wall MI are V_3 and V_4 and show ST segment elevation, T-wave inversion, and poor R-wave progression with deep Q waves. Leads opposite the affected area in an anterior wall myocardial infarction are II, III, and aVF and show depressed ST segments and tall R waves. See Figure 9-6 for anatomic location site and correlation to ECG electrode placement—please keep in mind that the red meshed area represents the anterior or front of the heart. See Figure 9-7 for a 12-lead ECG of an anterior wall myocardial infarction—pay particular attention to the changes in leads V_3 and V_4. Blockage of the diagonal branch of the left anterior descending artery affects the oxygenated blood supply to the right and left bundle branches and the ventricular septum. An anterior wall myocardial infarction may lead to second- or third-degree heart block, bundle branch blocks, irritability within the ventricles, and left ventricular dysfunction, resulting in heart failure. Occlusion of the left anterior descending artery above the diagonal branch in the left coronary artery can cause anterior wall damage as well as lateral and/or septal wall damage; therefore anterolateral or anteroseptal myocardial infarctions are a common occurrence. An occlusion of the left main coronary artery may be called "the widow-maker" due to its proclivity for advancing to cardiogenic shock and death. Blockage of the left anterior descending artery is considered particularly dangerous since this vessel supplies blood flow to a larger area of the heart than either the left circumflex artery or the right coronary artery and is primarily responsible for perfusing the left ventricle or powerhouse of the heart. Anterior wall myocardial infarctions tend to stimulate the sympathetic nervous system, resulting in tachycardia and hypertension.

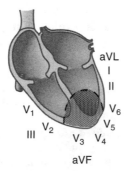

Figure 9-6   Anterior wall myocardial infarction anatomic site.

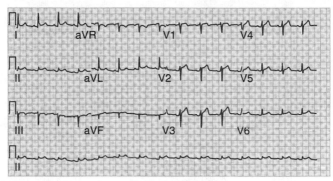

Figure 9-7   Anterior wall myocardial infarction.

Inferior Wall Myocardial Infarction

An inferior wall myocardial infarction develops when the right coronary artery becomes occluded in most individuals. In some individuals, the left circumflex artery will supply the inferior wall of the left ventricle via a posterior descending artery. Individuals with blood supply from the left circumflex artery are also at risk for a lateral wall or posterior wall MI if the proximal section of the artery is occluded. Leads facing the infarcted area of an inferior wall MI are II, III, and aVF, and show T-wave inversion, ST segment elevation, and pathologic Q waves. Leads opposite the affected area in an inferior wall myocardial infarction are I and aVL, and show ST segment depression. See Figure 9-8 for anatomic location site and correlation to ECG electrode placement. See Figure 9-9 for a 12-lead ECG of an inferior wall myocardial infarction—pay particular attention to the changes in leads II, III, and aVF. The right coronary artery supplies the SA node in 90% of individuals and the AV node in 50% of individuals. Logically then, the dysrhythmias that result from an inferior wall myocardial infarction are usually sinus bradycardia, sinoatrial arrest, and heart blocks. Premature ventricular contractions may occur from irritability of the cardiac tissue related to the release of enzymes from the dead necrotic tissue. Hypotension, elevated jugular vein distension, and crackles auscultated in the lungs are commonly related to the decreased cardiac output from the slow heart rate and are usually associated with infarction of the right ventricle as well as the inferior wall of the myocardium. Patients frequently complain of indigestion related to the proximity of the inferior wall of the myocardium to the diaphragm and deny chest pain when presenting with this infarction area.

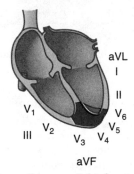

Figure 9-8   Inferior wall myocardial infarction anatomic site.

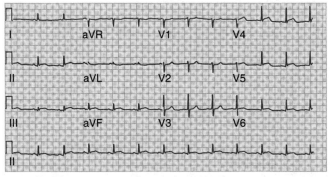

Figure 9-9   Inferior wall myocardial infarction.

Lateral Wall Myocardial Infarction

A lateral wall myocardial infarction develops when the left circumflex artery becomes occluded. Leads facing the affected area in a lateral wall MI are I, aVL, V_5, and V_6 and show ST segment elevation with Q waves in leads I and aVL. Many times, a pure lateral wall MI is overlooked, unless accompanied by an anterior or inferior wall MI. Leads opposite from the affected area in a lateral wall MI are II, III, and aVF, and show ST segment depression and tall T waves. See Figure 9-10 for anatomic location site and correlation to ECG electrode placement. See Figure 9-11 for a 12-lead ECG of a lateral wall myocardial infarction—pay particular attention to the changes in leads I, aVL, V_5, and V_6. Since a lateral wall MI is frequently accompanied by an anterior or inferior wall with more cardiac damage, the risk for complications of cardiogenic shock or heart failure increases dramatically. Conduction disturbances or heart blocks are commonly observed in lateral wall myocardial infarctions.

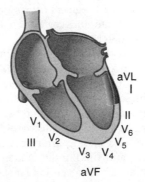

Figure 9-10   Lateral wall myocardial infarction anatomic site.

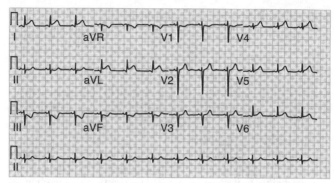

Figure 9-11   Lateral wall myocardial infarction.

Septal Wall Myocardial Infarction

A septal wall myocardial infarction develops when the septal branch of the left anterior descending artery becomes occluded. Leads facing the affected area in a septal wall MI are V_1, V_2, and V_3 and show T-wave inversion, ST segment elevation, and the elimination of an R wave. Leads opposite from the affected area in a septal wall MI are V_7, V_8, and V_9 seen in a 15-lead ECG and show ST segment depression. See Figure 9-12 for anatomic location site and correlation to ECG electrode placement. See Figure 9-13 for a 12-lead ECG of a septal wall myocardial infarction—pay particular attention to the changes in leads V_1 and V_2. A septal wall myocardial infarction is frequently seen in conjunction with an anterior wall myocardial infarction. The septal branch of the left anterior descending artery supplies the bundle of His and the bundle branches. Dysrhythmias that result from occlusion of the septal branch of the left anterior descending artery are Mobitz 2°, third-degree heart block, and the bundle branch blocks. In addition, the patient is at risk for a ventricular septal defect due to weakening of the myocardial wall from necrotic damage in the septum.

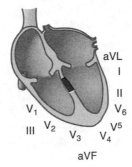

Figure 9-12   Septal wall myocardial infarction anatomic site.

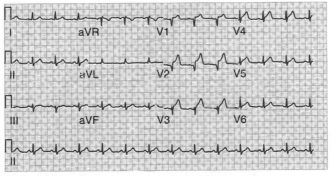

Figure 9-13   Septal wall myocardial infarction.

Posterior Wall Myocardial Infarction

A posterior wall myocardial infarction develops when either the posterior descending branch of the right coronary artery or the left circumflex artery becomes occluded. The right coronary artery typically supplies blood to the SA node, AV node, and bundle of His. Leads facing the affected area are V_7, V_8, and V_9 found in a 15-lead ECG and show ST segment elevation. A definitive diagnosis may require a 15-lead ECG. Leads opposite the affected area are V_1, V_2, V_3, and V_4, and show ST segment depression and tall R waves. See Figure 9-14 for anatomic location site and correlation to ECG electrode placement. See Figure 9-15 for a 12-lead ECG of a posterior wall myocardial infarction—pay particular attention to the changes in leads V_1, V_2, V_3, and V_4. Whenever ST segment depression is seen in V_1 to V_4, consider the possibility of a posterior wall myocardial infarction and obtain a 15-lead ECG. Posterior wall myocardial infarctions are frequently seen in conjunction with infarctions of either the lateral or inferior walls. Complications that originate from a posterior wall myocardial infarction are usually related to left ventricular dysfunction resulting in mild chronic heart failure and ventricular dysrhythmias.

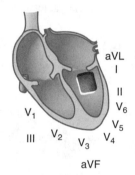

Figure 9-14   Posterior wall myocardial infarction anatomic site.

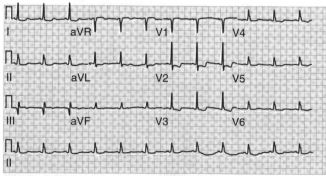

Figure 9-15   Posterior wall myocardial infarction.

MYOCARDIAL INFARCTION CARE MEASURES

The common phrase associated with the treatment of myocardial infarctions is "time is muscle." The longer the period of time that the cardiac muscle is in an oxygen-deficient state creates a higher likelihood for irreversible cardiac cell death. Early recognition and early treatment are critical to preserving cardiac muscle cells. The primary goal is to increase oxygen supply to the myocardium as quickly as possible through the use of methods that decrease oxygen demand of the coronary tissues, improve oxygen delivery to the tissues, and promote perfusion to the myocardium. If a myocardial infarction is suspected, a targeted history and physical assessment, drawing of serum cardiac markers, and attainment of 12-lead ECG are completed as quickly as possible. In fact, pre-hospital ECGs are now recommended to assist with decreasing time from emergency department admission to attainment of the first ECGs and to assist with decision-making on where to transport potential myocardial infarction patients. Timing is critical, as administration of fibrinolytics should be given within 30 minutes of admission to the emergency department or percutaneous coronary interventions implemented within 90 minutes of admission to the emergency department. Many smaller and rural hospital facilities do not offer percutaneous coronary interventional therapy. An ECG needs to be obtained within 10 minutes of entry to the emergency department and repeated in 1 to 2 hours. Other diagnostic tests that may be obtained include pulse oximetry, chest x-ray, complete blood count, electrolytes, and lipid profile.

While waiting for decisions on treatment, supplemental oxygen therapy is initiated, aspirin is administered, and nitroglycerin and/or morphine are given for pain. A method to remember the first four drugs to be administered is by the use of a mnemonic (MONA = morphine, oxygen, nitroglycerin, aspirin). Two large-bore intravenous catheters need to be inserted for immediate access and drug administration as needed. Oxygen is typically started at 2 to 4 L/min and titrated as needed to pulse oximetry of greater than 92%. Aspirin is a gold standard for prevention and treatment of acute myocardial infarction. Aspirin decreases

platelet aggregation, which decreases the risk of thrombus formation. If aspirin has not been taken prior to emergency room
admission, 162 to 325 mg of aspirin is given in a chewable format. Nitroglycerin is a direct vasodilator that dilates the venous
vascular bed, causing reduced preload, and to a lesser extent
dilates the coronary artery bed, which decreases afterload and
myocardial oxygen consumption. Nitroglycerin 0.4 mg sublingually may be given every 5 minutes up to three times if the chest
pain continues. For chest pain that continues beyond that point,
nitroglycerin or morphine intravenously may be given to decrease
the pain. When administering nitroglycerin sublingually or titrat-
ing the drug intravenously, intravenous access needs to be initiated, maintain systolic blood pressure greater than 90 mm Hg,
and avoid use of this drug if the patient has a right ventricular
infarct or has taken a phosphodiesterase inhibitor (Viagra, Cialis).
Morphine decreases pain and anxiety, leading to a reduction in
oxygen demand in the tissues. Two to four milligrams of morphine may be given intravenously every 5 minutes as needed to
eliminate pain as long as systolic blood pressure is maintained
greater than 90 mm Hg. Other possible medications include the
administration of anti-dysrhythmics, beta blockers, angiotensin-
converting enzyme inhibitors, and glycoprotein IIb/IIIa inhibitors.

Once initial actions have been taken to assess for a myocardial
infarction and while awaiting decision on treatment plan from
the cardiologist or emergency department physicians, actions
need to be taken to reduce oxygen demand, improve oxygen
supply, and improve cardiac tissue perfusion. Actions to reduce
oxygen demand include such measures as promoting rest, reducing pain with nitroglycerin and morphine, administration of beta
blockers, and administration of ACE inhibitors. Nitroglycerin
needs to be cautiously administered in patients with inferior wall
MIs related to the possibility of a right ventricular infarct and
higher risk for hypotension. Fluid boluses may need to be cautiously administered in inferior wall myocardial infarctions to
increase vascular volume to maintain blood pressure. Use of beta
blockers within 24 hours for patients with myocardial infarctions
is well supported within research as a measure to decrease

myocardial contractility and reduce cardiac workload. Beta blockers work by decreasing blood pressure thereby reducing afterload and cardiac workload and slowing heart rate, which increases ventricular filling time and increases cardiac output (Fact Sheet, 2005). Beta blocker administration has been shown to reduce reinfarction rates and further ischemia. Angiotensin-converting enzyme inhibitors (ACE inhibitors) are recommended to decrease afterload, thereby reducing cardiac workload and decreasing the incidence of ventricular remodeling. ACE inhibitors have been found to have a modest beneficial effect on decreasing mortality rates in all myocardial infarction patients (Danchin et al., 2006). Reducing afterload can be particularly useful in anterior wall MI patients who are experiencing hypertension. Oxygen supply to the cardiac tissue may be improved through administration of supplemental oxygen.

The third main thrust of care consists of methods to promote blood flow, which include such therapies as aspirin/glycoprotein IIb/IIIa inhibitors/thrombolytics, percutaneous transluminal coronary angioplasty (PTCA) with or without stent placement, coronary artery bypass graft (CABG), and intra-aortic balloon pump (IABP). Glycoprotein IIb/IIIa inhibitors work to prevent myocardial infarction and stent obstruction by blocking fibrinogen and von Willebrand factor from attaching to platelet receptors, thus preventing platelet aggregation. A meta-analysis review of research studies found that the combination of aspirin and clopidogrel therapy decreased the risk of cardiovascular crises, but significantly increased risk of bleeding in patients with acute coronary syndrome and post-percutaneous coronary interventions (Bowry et al, 2008). Thrombolytics may be administered to patients with ST segment elevation myocardial infarctions to convert plasminogen to plasmin, which is an enzyme that dissolves fibrin, resulting in the breakdown of a thrombus. Follow the agency's protocol for assessing for reperfusion therapy before administering thrombolytics. Thrombolytic therapy should be started within 30 minutes of entry to the emergency department if the patient is eligible for "clot busters" and angioplasty is not immediately available. Procedural therapies implemented to promote coronary artery blood flow include pacemakers, percutaneous coronary interventions, coronary artery bypass grafts, intra-aortic balloon pumping, and initiation of ventricular assist devices by physicians. Pacemakers may be needed, particularly with lateral and septal wall myocardial infarctions, to improve cardiac output and coronary artery blood flow if the patient experiences conduction disturbance heart blocks. Percutaneous coronary interventions should be implemented within 90 minutes of entry to the emergency department. Percutaneous coronary interventions include a variety of procedures designed to open the vessel at the occlusion using a balloon, a stent, or atherectomy. Coronary artery bypass graft is a surgical procedure that creates new routes for coronary artery blood to flow around the narrowed or occluded arteries to allow sufficient blood flow to reach the more distal areas of the heart.   Intra-aortic balloon pumps are temporary measures used either before, during, or after cardiac surgery (heart valve replacements, coronary artery bypass grafts, and cardiac transplants) to improve coronary artery blood flow and decrease cardiac workload through the inflation and deflation of a balloon threaded in by catheter to sit near the aortic arch. A ventricular assist device (VAD) is a measure to help a patient to survive until a cardiac transplant, or is used in severe heart failure patients who are not heart transplant candidates. The ventricular assist device is a mechanical pump located outside of the body; yet functions to pump the blood from the left ventricle to the aorta (left VAD) or from the right ventricle to the pulmonary artery (right VAD).

Myocardial Infarction Care Measures

- Obtain diagnostic information
  - History and physical assessment
  - Serum cardiac markers
  - ECG
  - Other tests

- Decrease oxygen demand of myocardial tissue
  — Promote rest
  — Treat pain with nitroglycerin and morphine
  — Administer beta blockers
- Improve oxygen delivery to myocardial tissue
  — Administer supplemental oxygen
- Improve blood flow to myocardial tissue
  — Administer aspirin
  — Administer thrombolytics (if PCI/CABG option unavailable)
  — Pacemaker
  — Percutaneous coronary interventions
  — Coronary artery bypass graft
  — Intra-aortic balloon pump/ventricular assist device

REFERENCES

Bowry AD, Brookhart MA, Choudhry NK. Meta-analysis of the efficacy and safety of clopidogrel plus aspirin as compared to antiplatelet monotherapy for the prevention of vascular events. *Am J Cardiol.* 2008;101:960–966.

Charpentier S. Diagnostic value of heart-fatty acid binding protein and ischemia modified albumin as biochemical markers on non-ST segment elevation acute coronary syndrome at the emergency room. U.S. National Institutes of Health, 2009. Retrieved on January 3, 2009 from http://clinicaltrials.gov/ct2/show/NCT00714298.

Danchin N, Cucherat M, Thuillez C, Durand E, Kadri Z, Steg PG. Angiotensin-converting enzyme inhibitors in patients with coronary artery disease and absence of heart failure or left ventricular systolic dysfunction: an overview of long-term randomized controlled trials. *Arch Int Med.* 2006;166:787–796.

Fact Sheet. Beta-blockers for acute myocardial infarction. Agency for Healthcare Research and Quality, 2005. Retrieved on January 3, 2009 from http://www.ahrq.gov/clinic/commitfact.htm.

Thygesen K, Alpert JS, White HD. Universal definition of myocardial infarction. *Circulation*. 2007;116:2634–2653. Retrieved on January 3, 2009 from http://circ.ahajournals.org/cgi/content/full/116/22/2634.

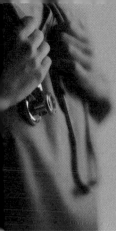

Chapter 10
PACEMAKERS

A pacemaker is a mechanical device that delivers an electrical impulse to stimulate the heart to depolarize. Pacemakers are composed of a pulse generator with a microchip that initiates an electrical impulse and manages the rate and intensity of the impulse. A second component of the pacemaker is a lead wire that connects the pulse generator to the cardiac muscle.

RATIONALE FOR PACEMAKER USE

Pacemakers may be used for a variety of dysrhythmias and heart failure (Table 10-1). The most common dysrhythmias requiring a pacemaker include bradydysrhythmias to increase the rate of the rhythm and therefore improve the cardiac output, second- and third-degree heart block to stimulate the ventricles to beat in synchrony with the atria to increase the cardiac output, and tachydysrhythmias to overdrive the atria and suppress the reentrant circuit. Frequently, pacemakers are needed immediately following cardiac surgery or after a myocardial infarction. Chronic heart failure and cardiomyopathy may interfere with the transmission of the electrical impulse through the heart, leading to the ventricles beating independent of each other and thus reducing cardiac output. Atriobiventricular pacing or resynchronization therapy can improve the contractility of the cardiac muscle by stimulating the ventricles to beat in synchrony.

Table 10-1   Rationale for Pacemaker Use

- Bradycardia
- Heart block
- Recurrent tachycardia
- Heart failure

TYPES

A single-chamber pacemaker has one electrode placed either in the right atria or ventricle to pace only one chamber in the heart, while a dual-chamber pacemaker has two electrodes with one placed in the atria and one placed in the ventricle to allow for coordination of functioning between the atria and ventricles (Table 10-2). Dual-chamber pacemakers are also called AV sequential pacemakers. A rate-responsive pacemaker has sensors within the pacemaker unit to adjust for changes in rate related to physical exercise, respirations, and physiologic changes. A rate-responsive pacemaker may be either a single-chamber or dual-chamber unit. An atriobiventricular pacer has one electrode in the right atria, a second electrode in the right ventricle, and a third electrode inserted through a vein, which innervates the left ventricle. The atriobiventricular pacer resynchronizes the heart to beat with more coordination between the chambers, leading to increased contractility and increased cardiac output, thus improving chronic heart failure. The atriobiventricular pacer, also known as cardiac resynchronization therapy (CRT), has been shown to decrease mortality and morbidity rates in patients with chronic heart failure (Cleland et al., 2005).

Table 10-2   Types of Pacemakers

- Single-chamber
- Dual-chamber
- Rate-responsive
- Atriobiventricular

LENGTH OF USE

Pacemakers may be employed on either a permanent or a temporary basis dependent on the patient's pathophysiologic state and projected need for the equipment. Permanent pacemakers are used for bradycardia, recurrent tachycardia, second- and third-degree heart block, and chronic heart failure. Temporary pacemakers are used for heart block after an inferior wall myocardial infarction, bradycardia, or tachydysrhythmias.

Permanent

A permanent pacemaker weighs approximately 1 ounce and is implanted underneath a clavicle on the patient's nondominant side or in the abdomen. The electrode lead wires are inserted via fluoroscopy into the subclavian vein and threaded into the right atria, right ventricle, or both depending on the type of pacemaker. The device is encased in titanium to reduce the possibility of rejection by the body. A lithium battery creates the electrical current necessary for generating the electronic signals. The battery generally lasts from 5 to 10 years.

Temporary

A temporary pacemaker is one that is used in an emergency when the patient's signs and symptoms deteriorate until the patient's crisis resolves or until a permanent pacemaker can be inserted. Temporary pacemakers are implemented via three main routes: transcutaneous, epicardial, and transvenous. For all forms of temporary pacing, close attention needs to be paid to keeping the settings at their intended values and avoiding accidental changes in measurements by patients, families, or health care providers.

ROUTES

Transcutaneous

Use of transcutaneous pacemakers has grown tremendously in the past few years. An electrode pad is placed anterior to the left of the sternum between the left nipple and the xiphoid process, and a second electrode pad is placed posterior on the patient's upper back right behind the pad on the chest (Fig. 10-1). Transcutaneous pads may be placed in an alternative

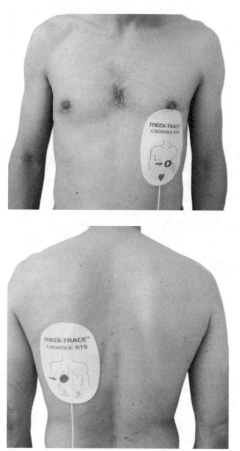

Figure 10-1   Anterior-posterior transcutaneous pacemaker pad placement.

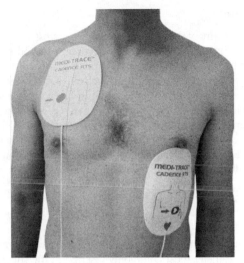

Figure 10-2   Chest transcutaneous pacemaker pad placement.

location of the right upper anterior chest with the second pad located anterior to the left of the sternum between the left nipple and the xiphoid process (Fig. 10-2). A pulse generator elicits an electrical impulse that travels from the skin to the cardiac muscle. During a cardiac arrest, the same pads may also be used for defibrillation if needed. Transcutaneous pads work well for emergencies due to their ease of application and ability to quickly establish a paced rhythm. Another advantage is the noninvasive nature of this method. Disadvantages of this method are more associated with long-term pacing such as effect of diaphoresis and loss of contact of the pad to the skin, patient discomfort, and activity restrictions. Transcutaneous pacing is not used in hypothermic bradycardia and flail chest.

Epicardial

A second form of temporary pacing is using an epicardial approach. Epicardial pacing is the typical method employed after cardiac surgery. This form of pacing is done by attaching lead wires to the epicardial surface of the heart during surgery, and bringing the wires to the chest wall distally to the incision. The lead wires may then be attached to the pulse generator. Lead wires are usually removed a few days after the cardiac surgery, when the patient no longer requires pacing. Epicardial pacing may be a more common pacing method for adolescents, children, and infants due to their anatomic structure.

Transvenous

A third form of temporary pacing is using a transvenous approach through a catheter most commonly inserted in the subclavian or internal jugular vein. The lead wires are threaded through the catheter into the right atrium or right ventricle, the pulse generator is then connected to the lead wires. A transvenous approach is more reliable than transcutaneous, but also more invasive.

SETTINGS

Programmable functions set on a pacemaker include rate (upper and lower limits), sensitivity, output, AV interval, and mode. Heart rates set on a pacemaker are usually from 60 to 80 bpm. A heart rate may be programmed into the pacemaker through calculating the heart rate in milliseconds. For example, a patient with a heart rate of 66 bpm would be programmed in a pacer as 909 milliseconds. Conversion of bpm to milliseconds is accomplished by dividing 60,000 by the heart rate. Through rate modulation, the heart rate may be programmed to increase or decrease by up to 5% of its immediately previous rhythm until the baseline is reached.

Diversity Impact

Pacemaker rates may be adjusted as children grow older and their baseline heart rates gradually decrease.

Two forms of sensitivity in pacemakers exist: demand and fixed. A demand pacemaker operates in synchrony with the patient's underlying heart rate. A demand pacemaker senses the patient's heartbeat and only initiates an electrical impulse when the patient's heart rate is lower than the preset pacemaker rate. The sensing threshold is measured in millivolts. A fixed rate pacemaker is asynchronous with the patient's underlying heart rate. A fixed rate pacemaker fires an electrical impulse without sensing the patient's underlying heart rate and may be used during cardiac arrest. Use of fixed rate pacemakers is limited due to the danger of a pacer spike landing on a T wave, sending the patient into ventricular fibrillation similar to an R-on-T phenomenon.

The output is the number of milliamperes needed in a pacer spike to initiate a contraction. The number of milliamperes may vary based on several factors, such as medications, which can change the electrical stimulus threshold; or embedding of the lead wire in scar tissue. The AV interval function in the pacemaker settings refers to the PR interval and reflects the amount of time the pacemaker waits after the atria are stimulated before sending an impulse to stimulate the ventricles.

The mode of the pacemaker is denoted by a five-letter international coding system that describes the function of the pacemaker. Pacemaker functions are coded for ease of interpretation by the North American Society of Pacing and Electrophysiology and the British Pacing and Electrophysiology Group (NASPE/BPEG). See Table 10-3. Although five functions are delineated through the use of the codes, the first three positions are the most frequently used in nursing clinical practice. Position I refers to the chamber(s) being paced and position II refers to the chamber(s) being sensed. Position III describes the action of the pacemaker when it senses the patient's underlying rhythm. Position IV reflects the rate modulation function, which allows for changes in heart rate dependent on the patient's exercise and activity. An adaptive rate mechanism uses piezoelectric crystal sensors to determine the patient's activity and then accelerate the patient's heart rate consistent with the activity needs. Position V depicts the presence of multisite pacing, absence of this form of pacing, or biatrial or biventricular pacing.

Table 10-3   The Revised NASPE/BPEG Generic Code for Antibradycardia Pacing

I	II	III	IV	V
Chamber(s) Paced	**Chamber(s) Sensed**	**Response to Sensing**	**Rate Modulation**	**Multisite Pacing**
0 = None	0 = None	0 = None	0 = None	0 = None
A = Atrium	A = Atrium	T = Triggered	R = Rate modulation	A = Atrium
V = Ventricle	V = Ventricle	I = Inhibited		V = Ventricle
D = Dual (A+V)	D = Dual (A+V)	D = Dual (T+I)		D = Dual (A+V)
S = Single (A or V)	S = Single (A or V)			

Last row of chambers paced and sensed are manufacturer's designation only.
Used with permission from Bernstein A, Daubert J, Fletcher R, et al. The revised NASPE/BPEG generic code for antibradycardia, adaptive-rate and multisite pacing. *Pacing Clinical Electrophysiology.* 25(2);2002,261.

Essentially, only two modes of pacemaker functioning are actively used today for single-chamber pacemakers. An atrial paced, sensed, and inhibited pacemaker (AAI) may be used for bradydysrhythmias when the rhythm initiates at the sinus node and an AV conduction disturbance does not exist (Fig. 10-3). A ventricular paced, sensed, and inhibited pacemaker (VVI) is frequently used for atrial fibrillation with a slow ventricular response rate (Fig. 10-4). Rate modulation is used when the sinus node does not function. Atrial and ventricular triggered action is infrequently used today for single-chamber pacemakers. Ventricular paced without sensing or responding to the sensing of a patient's underlying rhythm (VVO) has limited use, but may be seen during surgery when electrocautery is used.

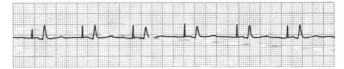

Figure 10-3   AAI pacing.

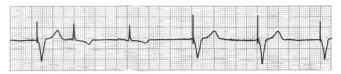

Figure 10-4   VVI pacing.

Dual-chamber pacemakers or AV sequential pacing are usually more useful to improve cardiac output and decrease risk of heart failure. The DOO mode of pacing occurs when a magnet is placed on the pacemaker, which makes the pacemaker pace, but eliminates sensing of the patient's rhythm. DOO mode can be used diagnostically or to avoid inappropriate sensing and electromagnetic interference. An AV sequential pacemaker has a DVI setting to allow for sensing of spontaneous QRS complexes. In the DVI setting, the pacemaker paces the atria and then the ventricles when the ventricles do not spontaneously create a QRS complex. DDD mode of pacing is the most frequently used mode in permanent pacemakers. The dual pacing, sensing, and responding to sensing with both triggering and inhibiting actions characteristic of DDD pacing are used for left ventricular dysfunction, heart failure, and AV blocks (Fig. 10-5).

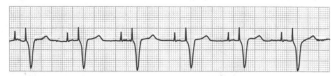

Figure 10-5   DDD pacing.

PACEMAKER INTERPRETATION CRITERIA

A paced rhythm varies based on the location site of the pacemaker and demand or fixed rate functioning. The characteristic finding in any paced rhythm is a pacemaker spike. A pacemaker spike is a vertical line on the ECG that should be located just prior to a P wave for atrial pacing and just prior to a QRS complex for ventricular pacing. The pacer spike indicates that the pacemaker has discharged an electrical impulse to the heart muscle to depolarize one of the heart chambers and initiate a contraction.

Pacemaker Interpretation Criteria

1. Rhythm—Varies based on demand or fixed rate functioning
   A. Demand—Irregular unless heart being paced 100% of the time
   B. Fixed rate—Regular
2. Rate:
   A. Demand—Fluctuates based on patient's underlying rhythm, but no less than preset pacemaker rate
   B. Fixed rate—Consistent at predetermined pacemaker rate

3. P wave:
   A. Atrial pacer—P wave follows each atrial pacer spike
   B. Ventricular pacer—No P waves or SA node P waves unrelated to QRS complexes
   C. AV sequential pacer—P wave follows each atrial pacer spike
   D. Biventricular pacer—P wave follows each atrial pacer spike
4. PRI:
   A. Atrial pacer—Constant PRI
   B. Ventricular pacer—None
   C. AV sequential pacer—Constant PRI
   D. Biventricular pacer—Constant PRI
5. QRS I:
   A. Atrial pacer—Less than 0.12 sec, unless patient has BBB
   B. Ventricular pacer—Wide bizarre, QRS complex; greater than 0.12 sec and follows each ventricular pacer spike
   C. AV sequential pacer—Wide bizarre, QRS complex, greater than 0.12 sec and follows each ventricular pacer spike
   D. Biventricular pacer—Wide bizarre, QRS complex; greater than 0.12 sec and follows each ventricular pacer spike

INTERFERENCE WITH PACEMAKER FUNCTION

Several electrical and magnetic sources may interfere with the pacemaker function, causing pacemaker rates to change, preventing electrical output initiating beats, and damaging the pulse generator (Table 10-4). Patients need to be educated about electromagnetic sources and counseled on increasing their awareness of their physiologic states when near a source. Occupational evaluation of sources within work environments may identify potential issues such as arc welding equipment, power generators, and devices with magnets. Magnetic resonance imaging (MRI) may interfere with the pacing and require reprogramming of the pacemaker after the MRI is performed. A benefit-risk analysis needs to be performed before an MRI is scheduled for the patient with a pacemaker. Diagnostic x-rays may be obtained without issue; yet radiation therapy may interfere with the pacemaker circuits. Covering the pacemaker with a lead apron when able, monitoring an ECG during radiation treatment, and frequent pulse generator checks after treatment are advised to promote safe pacemaker function. A transcutaneous electrical nerve stimulator (TENS) unit used to control pain may occasionally and briefly inhibit unipolar pacing, which will require pacemaker reprogramming. Radiofrequency ablation used to treat dysrhythmias rarely interferes with pacemaker function, but function needs to be evaluated after this treatment. Extracorporeal shock wave lithotripsy (ESWL) used to dissolve renal stones may require pacemaker reprogramming immediately after treatment and evaluation of pacemaker functioning for several months after treatment. Patients with abdominally placed pacemakers needing ESWL need to consider alternative therapy for treatment of renal lithiasis. Dental procedures may increase pacer rates. Short-wave and microwave diathermy used as a form of heat therapy may irreparably damage the pulse generator, and alternative treatments should be sought. Cell phone companies are tinkering with new frequencies that may interfere with functioning. Currently, cell phones in the United States use less than 3 watts and do not interfere with pacemaker functioning. Airport screening devices do not disturb pacemaker function, but may sense the pacemaker and alarm, requiring individuals to be "wanded" rather than walking through the screener. The wand or handheld screening device should not be placed over the top of the pacemaker. Retail anti-theft devices and electronic surveillance equipment may need to be avoided if the patient experiences symptoms. Initially, iPods were considered to be possible electromagnetic interference sources that could affect pacemaker function. A recent study by the FDA found no interference effects of iPods on pacemaker functioning (Bassen, 2008).

Table 10-4   Sources Interfering with Pacemaker Function

- Occupational and hobby hazards
  - Arc welding
  - Power generating equipment
  - Magnets
- Health care hazards
  - Magnetic resonance imaging
  - Radiation therapy
  - TENS unit
  - Radiofrequency ablation
  - Extracorporeal shock wave lithotripsy
  - Dental procedures
  - Shortwave and microwave diathermy
- Lifestyle technologies
  - Cell phones
  - Airport screening
  - Anti-theft devices

PACEMAKER MALFUNCTION

Four main types of ECG changes may occur with pacemaker malfunction: failure to pace, failure to capture, failure to sense, and oversensing.

Failure to Pace

Failure to pace is the lack of pacemaker spikes in the patient with a slower heart rate than the pacemaker setting and a return of the patient's previous rhythm. In this instance, the pacemaker is failing to generate an electrical impulse to stimulate the heart (Fig. 10-6). Causes of failure to pace include battery malfunction, dislodgement of the lead, fractured wire, disconnected wire, or pulse generator failure. The ECG finding is an absence of a pacer spike when one should have occurred. The patient may exhibit signs and symptoms of decreased cardiac output from bradycardia, which can deteriorate into asystole. Treatment is to identify the cause of failure to pace and intervene as needed, which can involve something as simple as a battery change to checking all connections on a temporary pacemaker to complete replacement of the pacemaker.

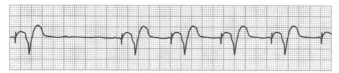

Figure 10-6   Failure to pace.

Failure to Capture

Failure to capture is the presence of a pacer spike located in the appropriate position, but lacking enough "juice" or milliamperes to cause depolarization in the heart muscle. For an atrial pacer with failure to capture, a pacer spike is seen without a P wave following the spike. For a ventricular pacer with failure to capture, a pacer spike is seen without a QRS complex following the spike (Fig. 10-7). Causes of failure to capture include battery malfunction, dislodgement of the lead, fractured wire, myocardial perforation, a low milliampere setting, acidosis, and electrolyte imbalances. The patient may exhibit signs of a cardiac arrest such as pulselessness and asystole. Again, treatment revolves around identifying the cause and intervening as needed, such as obtaining a chest x-ray to determine lead dislodgement, fractured wire, or myocardial perforation; correcting metabolic disturbances of acidosis or electrolyte imbalances; positioning the patient on his or her side and adjusting milliampere settings to achieve capture.

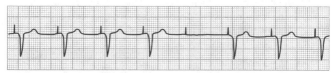

Figure 10-7   Failure to capture.

Failure to Sense

Failure to sense is the inappropriate firing of the pacemaker at any point in the cardiac cycle. Pacer spikes can occur anywhere on the ECG and do not necessarily precede a P wave or QRS complex (Fig. 10-8). Causes of failure to sense include depleted battery states, application of magnets to the pacemaker, dislodgement of leads, mode of pacemaker function, edema or scarring raising the pacing threshold after a myocardial infarction, electrolyte imbalances, or drug interactions. Failure to sense in a VOO or DOO mode setting is a programmable limitation of that mode of pacing. For synchronous pacing, failure to sense is dangerous, particularly if the pacer spike is landing on the T wave, which may precipitate ventricular fibrillation. The patient may exhibit palpitations. Care for the patient with failure to sense revolves around determining the cause and treating it, such as removing electromagnetic interference, replacing the pulse generator battery, or adjusting the sensitivity dial.

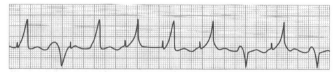

Figure 10-8   Failure to sense.

Oversensing

Oversensing is the misinterpretation by the pacemaker that muscle movement or other activities are actually cardiac depolarization. As a result, the pacemaker does not fire when the patient needed the electrical stimulus to initiate cardiac depolarization. On the ECG, the heart rate is noted to be lower than the rate set on the pacemaker (Fig. 10-9). Causes of oversensing include electromagnetic interference, hyperkalemia with large T waves, muscle movements of shivering or seizures, programmed pacemaker rate set too low, and battery failure. The patient may exhibit signs and symptoms of reduced cardiac output due to the decreased heart rate. Care measures to rectify an oversensing problem may include changing the sensitivity, increasing the rate set on the pacemaker, verifying grounding of electrical sources, replacing the battery, and treating hyperkalemia, shivering, or seizures.

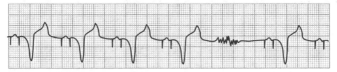

Figure 10-9   Oversensing.

CARE MEASURES AFTER PERMANENT PACEMAKER INSERTION

After a permanent pacemaker has been inserted, assessment of the patient is necessary to evaluate the effectiveness of the unit. Patient assessment involves observing for symptoms of decreased cardiac output, determining the presence of a pacer spike and resultant P or QRS waves dependent on the mode of pacing, and evaluating for the presence of pacemaker malfunction including failure to pace, failure to capture, failure to sense, and oversensing. Mild analgesics may be prescribed for the first couple of days after a permanent pacemaker has been inserted to promote comfort. Patients need to be instructed to keep manufacturer pacemaker information with them at all times, how to take their pulse, when to call their cardiologist, initial activity restrictions, and sources of electromagnetic interference. For the first 4 to 6 weeks after pacemaker insertion, activity restrictions include preventing arm movement above head and out to side and no lifting greater than 5 pounds with arm on side of pacemaker insertion to allow for stabilization of lead wire into cardiac tissue. Tennis, golf, and swimming need to be avoided for the first 6 weeks. Patients will need follow-up appointments for the rest of their life, usually about every 6 to 12 months to evaluate pacemaker function and battery life. A cardiologist may determine pacemaker function by applying a magnet to the pacemaker. Use of a magnet over a pacemaker forces the pacemaker into asynchronous pacing, which allows for evaluation of capture, chambers being paced, and battery life. Keep transcutaneous pacing equipment nearby when magnets are used in case of malfunctioning of the pacemaker. Before using a magnet, always read the manufacturer's information to validate that the device inserted in the patient is not an implantable cardioverter-defibrillator, as the magnet will inactivate the cardioversion-defibrillation activity. The life of the battery depends on the number of millivolts needed to capture the rhythm, presence of single versus dual chamber pacing, and the amount of time the patient spends in a paced rhythm on a daily basis.

Care Measures after Permanent Pacemaker Insertion

- Assess the patient for syncope, dyspnea, confusion, hiccups, and bradycardia/tachycardia.
- Medicate for discomfort for first couple of days after procedure with mild analgesics.
- Provide the manufacturer's card to the patient and instruct to keep in wallet.
- Teach the patient how to take his or her own pulse.
- Instruct to call cardiologist if pulse drops below set pacemaker rate.
- Educate the patient on electromagnetic sources and actions to take.
- Teach the patient about initial activity restrictions.
- Explain the necessity for follow-up appointments for the rest of his or her life.

CARE MEASURES AFTER TEMPORARY PACEMAKER PLACEMENT

Hiccups and twitching in synchrony with the pacer spikes may occur due to stimulation from the pacemaker. Assessment for lead wire perforation, cardiac tamponade, or pneumothorax is critical and can be life-threatening if not assessed and treated early. Symptoms of cardiac tamponade include dyspnea, hypotension, tachycardia, syncope, and jugular vein distension. Clinical symptoms of pneumothorax are dyspnea and diminished lung sounds. Chest x-rays are ordered after insertion of transvenous and epicardial pacemakers to verify placement and determine presence of pneumothorax. Electrocardiograms are obtained before and after temporary pacemaker placement, with every pacemaker setting change, and usually about once a day if the patient is stable. When using a transcutaneous pacemaker, make sure that the machine is set for pacing and not defibrillation, and expect the physician to order settings of 60 to 70 bpm. The number of milliamperes is determined by increasing the mA setting until capture is reached, and then adjusting the setting 20 mA higher than where capture was achieved. Discomfort from the pacing stimulus may be treated with mild analgesics. Microshocks may occur with electrical equipment that is not grounded properly. With epicardial pacer wires, the risk for microshocks may be decreased by wrapping with nonconductive tape the ends of the lead wires that attach to the pulse generator when the pacemaker is not in use. Gloves need to be worn when working with the exposed lead wires. The lead wires should be kept separate from each other and wrapped individually during dressing changes. The external pulse generator box needs to have a plastic cover to prevent accidental changing of settings. Usually the external pulse generator box is suspended on an intravenous pole or pinned to the sheets. An extra external pulse generator and battery need to be kept on the unit in case of failure of the unit being used on the patient. Use of arms away from body or abducted positioning should be prevented, and care needs to be taken when getting the patient out of bed to prevent dislodgement of lead wires, especially when using either a transvenous or epicardial approach to pacing.

Care Measures with a Temporary Pacemaker

- Assess the patient for syncope, dyspnea, confusion, hiccups, and bradycardia/tachycardia.
- Assess for twitching of chest muscles and medicate for comfort as needed.
- Verify the patient's pacemaker settings: rate, mA, sensitivity, pacing mode, presence of pacer spike.
- Assess for malfunctioning of the pacemaker and report to the cardiologist as needed: failure to pace, failure to capture, failure to sense, and oversensing.
- Obtain ECGs and chest x-rays as needed.
- Treat discomfort with mild analgesics.
- Validate grounding of all electrical equipment within patient's room.
- Prevent accidental pacemaker setting changes.
- Reposition the patient carefully, as turning may dislodge the lead wires.
- Instruct the patient to call for assistance before getting out of bed.

IMPLANTABLE CARDIOVERTER-DEFIBRILLATOR (ICD)

An Implantable Cardioverter-Defibrillator (ICD) is used to treat bradycardia, recurrent, sustained ventricular tachycardia, or ventricular fibrillation. The device can sense when the patient develops ventricular tachycardia or ventricular fibrillation and deliver a shock to convert the patient back to normal sinus rhythm. Newer ICDs can perform overdrive pacing for tachy-dysrhythmias, pacing for bradydysrhythmias, and biventricular pacing. Most of the time, ICDs are used in patients whose dys-rhythmias have been unable to be controlled with medications, catheter ablation, or surgery. Similar to permanent pacemakers, an ICD may be inserted during open heart surgery or through vessels to cardiovert, defibrillate, or pace the heart. An ICD is composed of lead wires positioned either endocardially or epi-cardially, which are connected to a pulse generator. Although slightly larger than the pulse generator for a permanent pace-maker, the placement is identical within the body; either under the skin below the left clavicle or in the abdomen. When the ICD discharges for cardioversion, the patient may feel like he or she is being punched in the chest. If the heart rate remains ele-vated, the ICD will discharge at a higher voltage in an attempt to defibrillate the patient's rhythm. When the ICD discharges for defibrillation, the patient may fall to the ground. During cardioversion and defibrillation, the spike seen on telemetry is larger than a spike seen during pacing activity. If the patient develops a dysrhythmia requiring cardiopulmonary resuscita-tion, begin CPR and deliver defibrillation as needed. Placement of the defibrillation electrodes is preferred in the anterior-pos-terior location to avoid placement over the pulse generator of the ICD. See Figure 10-1. If the ICD defibrillates when the health care provider has contact with the chest, the provider may feel the electrical shock. Gloves are recommended during CPR activities to decrease electrical conduction into the health care provider. Similar to permanent pacemakers, activity within the first 24 hours after ICD placement is restricted and then gradu-ally increased as tolerated. Necessary patient education includes carrying of ICD information at all times, warning of possibility of electrical interference from equipment, and the need to inform health care providers of the device, particularly before CT and MRI scans. The family needs to be educated on the use of an ICD device, plus initiation of the 911 emergency response system and performance of CPR in case of ICD failure.

REFERENCES

Bassen H. Low frequency magnetic emissions and resulting induced voltages in a pacemaker by iPod portable music players. *Biomed Eng OnLine*. 2008;7. Retrieved on February 21, 2009 from http://www.biomedical-engineering-online.com/content/7/1/7.

Bernstein A, Camm A, Fisher J, et al. North American Society of Pacing and Electrophysiology/British Pacing and Electrophysiology Group policy statement. The NASPE/ BPEG defibrillator code. *Pacing Clin Electrophysiol*. 1993;16: 1776–1780.

Bernstein A, Daubert J, Fletcher R, et al. The revised NASPE/BPEG generic code for antibradycardia, adaptive-rate, and multisite pacing. North American Society of Pacing and Electrophysiology/ British Pacing and Electrophysiology Group. *Pacing Clin Electrophysiol*. 2002;25:260–264.

Cleland J, Daubert J, Erdmann E, et al. The effect of cardiac resynchronization on morbidity and mortality in heart failure. *N Engl J Med*. 2005;352:1539–1549.

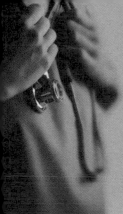

BRADYCARDIA ALGORITHM

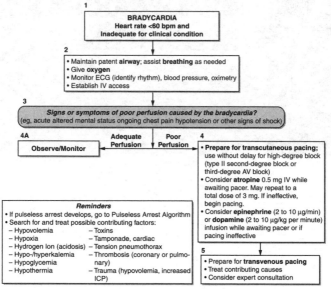

1

> **BRADYCARDIA**
> Heart rate <60 bpm and
> Inadequate for clinical condition

2

- Maintain patent **airway**; assist **breathing** as needed
- Give **oxygen**
- Monitor ECG (identify rhythm), blood pressure, oximetry
- Establish IV access

3

> *Signs or symptoms of poor perfusion caused by the bradycardia?*
> (eg, acute altered mental status ongoing chest pain hypotension or other signs of shock)

4A — Adequate Perfusion → **Observe/Monitor**

Poor Perfusion ↓

4

- **Prepare for transcutaneous pacing;** use without delay for high-degree block (type II second-degree block or third-degree AV block)
- Consider **atropine** 0.5 mg IV while awaiting pacer. May repeat to a total dose of 3 mg. If ineffective, begin pacing.
- Consider **epinephrine** (2 to 10 μg/min) or **dopamine** (2 to 10 μg/kg per minute) infusion while awaiting pacer or if pacing ineffective

5

- Prepare for **transvenous pacing**
- Treat contributing causes
- Consider expert consultation

Reminders

- If pulseless arrest develops, go to Pulseless Arrest Algorithm
- Search for and treat possible contributing factors:
  - Hypovolemia
  - Hypoxia
  - Hydrogen Ion (acidosis)
  - Hypo-/hyperkalemia
  - Hypoglycemia
  - Hypothermia
  - Toxins
  - Tamponade, cardiac
  - Tension pneumothorax
  - Thrombosis (coronary or pulmonary)
  - Trauma (hypovolemia, increased ICP)

BRADYCARDIA ALGORITHM

Reprinted with Permission: 2005 American Heart Association Guidelines for Cardiopulmonary Resuscitation and Emergency Cardiovascular Care, Circulation. 2005;112(suppl IV) ©2005, American Heart Association, Inc.

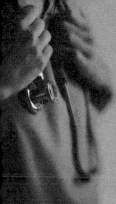

Appendix B

ACLS TACHYCARDIA ALGORITHM

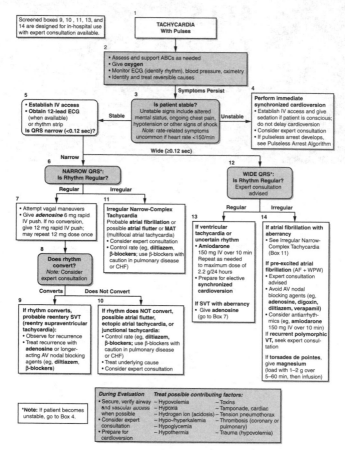

ACLS TACHYCARDIA ALGORITHM

Reprinted with Permission: 2005 American Heart Association Guidelines for Cardiopulmonary Resuscitation and Emergency Cardiovascular Care, Circulation. 2005;112(suppl IV) ©2005, American Heart Association, Inc.

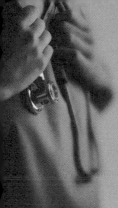

Appendix C

ACLS PULSELESS ARREST ALGORITHM

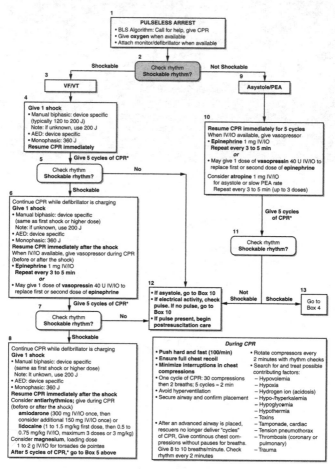

ACLS PULSELESS ARREST ALGORITHM

Reprinted with Permission: 2005 American Heart Association Guidelines for Cardiopulmonary Resuscitation and Emergency Cardiovascular Care, Circulation. 2005;112(suppl IV) ©2005, American Heart Association, Inc.

Index

Note: Page numbers referencing figures are followed by an "*f*;" page numbers referencing tables are followed by a "*t*."

A

A flutter (*see* Atrial flutter)
AAI (atrial paced, sensed, and inhibited pacemaker), 288–289
Aberrantly conducted premature atrial contraction, 52*f*
Absolute refractory period, 4
Accelerated idioventricular rhythm (AIVR):
   assessment of, 134
   care measures for, 136–137
   causes of, 133–134
   heart rate and, 213
   interpretation criteria, 135–136
   overview, 133
Accelerated junctional rhythm (AJR):
   assessment of, 95
   care measures for, 97
   causes of, 94–95
   interpretation criteria, 96
   overview, 94
ACE inhibitors (angiotensin-converting enzyme inhibitors), 277
Acetylcholine, 6
Acidosis, 222
ACLS pulseless arrest algorithm, 308
ACLS tachycardia algorithm, 306
Acute pancreatitis, 230
Acute phase, MI, 252
Adenosine, 37, 70, 106, 110–111
Advanced Mobitz block, 174
AED (automatic external defibrillator), 308
AF (*see* Atrial fibrillation)
Afterdepolarizations, 24, 47
Afterload, 5
Agonal rhythm, 129
AIVR (*see* Accelerated idioventricular rhythm)
AJR (*see* Accelerated junctional rhythm)

Albumin:
   effect on total serum calcium levels, 238
   magnesium and, 229
Albuterol, 64, 226, 227*t*
Alcohol:
   hypokalemia and, 216
   hypomagnesemia and, 230
Alkalosis, 216
Aminoglycosides, 230
Amiodarone:
   premature ventricular contraction, 127–128
   pulseless arrest, 308
   tachycardia, 306
   ventricular fibrillation, 150
   ventricular tachycardia, 142
   Wolff–Parkinson–White syndrome, 111
Analgesics, 296
Anatomy of heart, 5*f*
Angina pectoris, 255,256*t*, 262
Angiotensin-converting enzyme inhibitors (ACE inhibitors), 277
Antegrade depolarization, 84, 89, 94, 98
Anterior wall myocardial infarction, 267–269
Anterior-posterior transcutaneous pacemaker pads, 284*f*
Antibradycardia pacing, 288*t*
Anti-coagulation therapy, 77
Antiarrhythmics, 308
Antidysrhythmics:
   accelerated idioventricular rhythm, 136
   atrial flutter and, 70
   converting rhythm, 143
   idioventricular rhythm, 132
Antithrombotic therapy, 78*t*
Anxiety, 255
Artifacts, ECG, 24–25, 143
Aspirin, 78, 275–276

310   Index

Asymptomatic Mobitz block, 176
Asymptomatic rhythm, PVC, 127
Asynchronous pacing, 297
Asystole:
    assessment of, 158–159
    care measures for, 160
    causes of, 157–158
    interpretation criteria, 159
    overview, 156–157
AT (see Atrial tachycardia)
Atheromatous plaques, 252
Atrial bradycardia, 55
Atrial fibrillation (AF):
    assessment of, 74
    care measures for, 76–79
    causes of, 73
    interpretation criteria, 75–76
    overview, 71–73
    tachycardia, 306
Atrial flutter (A flutter):
    assessment of, 67
    care measures for, 69–71
    causes of, 66–67
    interpretation criteria, 68–69
    overview, 65
    P′ waves, 197
Atrial paced, sensed, and inhibited
        pacemaker (AAI), 288–289
Atrial regularity, 15
Atrial rhythms, 47–82
    atrial fibrillation: assessment of, 74
        care measures for, 76–79
        causes of, 73
        interpretation criteria, 75–76
        overview, 71–73
    atrial flutter: assessment of, 67
        care measures for, 69–71
        causes of, 66–67
        interpretation criteria, 68–69
        overview, 65
    atrial tachycardia: assessment of,
        60–61
        care measures for, 63–64
        causes of, 59–60
        interpretation criteria, 61–63
        overview, 58–59
    comparison of, 80–81
    differentiating, 191t
    overview, 47
    premature atrial contractions:
        assessment of, 49–50
        care measures for, 53–54
        causes of, 48–49

Atrial rhythms, premature atrial
        contractions: assessment of (Cont.):
        interpretation criteria, 50–53
        overview, 48
    wandering atrial pacemaker:
        assessment of, 56
        care measures for, 57–58
        causes of, 55–56
        interpretation criteria, 56–57
        overview, 55
Atrial tachycardia (AT):
    assessment of, 60–61
    care measures for, 63–64
    causes of, 59–60
    interpretation criteria, 61–63
    overview, 58–59
    P′ waves, 197
    premature atrial contraction and, 51
Atriobiventricular pacing, 281–282
Atrioventricular (AV) heart blocks,
        163–188
    bundle branch block: assessment of,
        183
        care measures for, 185
        causes of, 182
        interpretation criteria, 183–185
        overview, 180–182
    comparison of, 186–187
    differentiating, 191t
    first-degree: assessment of, 165
        care measures for, 166–167
        causes of, 164–165
        interpretation criteria, 165–166
        overview, 163–164
    second-degree: Mobitz 2°, 172–176
        Wenckebach, 167–171
    third-degree: assessment of,
        177–178
        care measures for, 180
        causes of, 177
        interpretation criteria, 178–179
        overview, 176–177
Atrioventricular (AV) node, 8
Atropine:
    accelerated idioventricular rhythm, 136
    asystole, 160
    bradycardia treatment, 304
    pulseless arrest, 308
    pulseless electrical activity, 155
    sinus bradycardia and, 31–32
Augmented leads, 9
Automatic external defibrillator (AED),
        142

Automaticity:
    cardiac cells, 2
    enhanced, 47, 66
    sinoatrial arrest and, 42
AV (atrioventricular) node, 8
AV dissociation, 130
AV heart blocks (see Atrioventricular
        heart blocks)
AV nodal reentricular tachycardia
        (AVNRT):
    assessment of, 104–105
    care measures for, 106–107
    causes of, 103–104
    interpretation criteria, 105
    overview, 102–103
AV reentrant tachycardia (AVRT):
    assessment of, 109
    care measures for, 111–112
    causes of, 108–109
    interpretation criteria, 109–111
    overview, 107–108
AV sequential pacemakers, 282, 289
AVNRT (see AV nodal reentrant
        tachycardia)

B
Bachmann bundle, 7
Basic life-support (BLS) protocol, 142
BBB (see Bundle branch block)
Beta blockers:
    atrial fibrillation, 77
    atrial flutter and, 70
    myocardial infarction, 277
    potassium and, 222
    premature ventricular contraction,
        127–128
    Wolff–Parkinson–White syndrome, 111
Bigeminal premature ventricular
        contractions, 123f
Bisphosphonates, 248
BLS (basic life-support) protocol, 142
Body temperature, 34
Bradycardia, 193–196, 304
    (See also Sinus bradycardia)
Bradycardia algorithm, 304
Bradycardic rhythms, 194–195t
Bundle branch block (BBB):
    assessment of, 183
    care measures for, 185
    causes of, 182
    interpretation criteria, 183–185
    overview, 180–182
    QRS interval and, 47

Bundle branches, 8
Bundle of His, 8

C
CABG (coronary artery bypass graft),
        277–278
Calcitonin, 238, 248
Calcitriol, 238, 244
Calcium:
    dietary sources of, 243
    hypercalcemia: assessment of,
        245–246
        care measures for, 247–248
        causes of, 244–245
        interpretation criteria,
            246–247
        overview, 243–244
    hypocalcemia: assessment of,
        240–241
        care measures for, 242–243
        causes of, 239–240
        interpretation criteria, 242
        overview, 239
    overview, 237–238
Calcium channel blockers, 77, 111
Calcium chloride, 243
Calcium gluconate:
    hyperkalemia and, 227t
    hypermagnesemia and, 237
    hypocalcemia and, 243
Calipers, 16
Cancer, 244, 248
Cardiac cells:
    automaticity, 2
    conductivity, 3
    contractility, 3
    excitability, 2–3
    refractoriness, 3–4
Cardiac output, 5, 192t
Cardiac regulation, 6
Cardiac resynchronization therapy
        (CRT), 185, 282
Cardiac tamponade, 298
Cardiac telemetry monitoring, 220
Cardiopulmonary resuscitation (CPR),
        143, 308
Cardiovascular blood flow, 5–6
Cardioversion, 70, 306
Carotid sinus massage, 106
Catecholamines:
    hypomagnesemia and, 230
    sinus tachycardia and, 33
    vasopressin and, 144

Catheter ablation, 64, 70, 111
Cation-exchange resins, 226
CHB (complete heart block)
  (*see* Third-degree heart block)
Chelating agents, 248
Chest pain, 254–255, 256*t*, 262–263
Children:
  atrial tachycardia in, 63
  epicardial pacing in, 286
  junctional tachycardia in, 101
  respiratory sinus dysrhythmia in, 39
  sinus bradycardia and, 29
  Wenckebach block in, 168
Chronic atrial fibrillation, 77
Chronic heart failure, 74
Chvostek sign, 241*f*
Cisplatin chemotherapy, 230
Citrate, 239
CK-MB mass, 258*t*
Coarse atrial fibrillation, 75
Coarse fibrillatory waves, 150
Coarse ventricular fibrillation, 148*f*
Compensatory pause, 125*f*
Complete AV block, 163
Complete heart block (CHB)
  (*see* Third-degree heart block)
Conduction pathway:
  accelerated idioventricular rhythm, 133*f*
  accelerated junctional rhythm, 94*f*
  asystole, 156*f*
  atrial fibrillation, 72*f*
  atrial flutter, 65*f*
  atrial tachycardia, 59*f*
  AV nodal reentrant tachycardia, 103*f*
  fetal, 108
  first-degree heart block, 164*f*
  heart, 7*f*
  idioventricular rhythm, 129*f*
  junctional escape rhythm, 89*f*
  junctional tachycardia, 98*f*
  left bundle branch block, 181*f*
  premature atrial contraction, 48*f*
  premature ventricular contractions,
    118*f*
  pulseless electrical activity, 152*f*
  right bundle branch block, 181*f*
  second-degree heart block, 167*f*, 172
  sinoatrial arrest, 41*f*
  third-degree heart block, 176*f*
  ventricular fibrillation, 146*f*
  ventricular tachycardia, 137*f*
  wandering atrial pacemaker, 55*f*
  Wolff–Parkinson–White syndrome, 108*f*

Conductivity, 3
Constipation, 31
Contiguous leads, 260, 261*t*
Contractility, 3
Controlled atrial fibrillation, 75*f*
Coronary artery bypass graft (CABG),
    277–278
Corticosteroids, 248
Countdown methods, 17–18*t*
  large box, 18–19
  "quick and dirty," 19
  small box, 18
Couplets, 122–123, 124*f*
CPR (cardiopulmonary resuscitation),
    143, 308
CRT (cardiac resynchronization
    therapy), 185, 282

D
DDD mode, pacing, 289–290
Defibrillation, 149–150, 308
Delta wave, 21, 109, 180, 183
Demand pacemakers, 287
Depolarization:
  antegrade and retrograde, 84, 89,
    94, 98
  defined, 1–2
Diabetes mellitus:
  atrial flutter and, 66
  potassium and, 222
Diarrhea, 216
Diastole, shortened, 60
Dietary sources:
  calcium, 243
  magnesium, 233
Differentiation of rhythms:
  bradycardia versus tachycardia,
    193–198
  extrasystolic beats, 192–193
  by location site, 190–191
  narrow versus wide QRS,
    207–213
  pulseless rhythms, 213–214
  regular versus irregular, 198–207
Digibind, 136
Digoxin:
  accelerated junctional rhythm, 94
  atrial flutter, 70
  automaticity and, 55
  contractility and, 3
  junctional tachycardia, 98
  PJCs and, 84–85
  toxicity, 61

Diltiazem, 3, 70
Dofetilide, 70
DOO mode, pacing, 289, 295
Dopamine, 304
Doppler ultrasound, 154
Dual-chamber pacemakers, 282, 289
"Dying" heart, 129
Dysrhythmias:
    basis of, 23–24
    hypokalemia and, 218
    inferior wall myocardial infarction,
        269
    septal branch myocardial infarction,
        272

E
Early repolarization, 1
ECG (electrocardiogram):
    artifacts, 24–25, 143
    interpretation method:
        differentiation of rhythms,
            189–214
        overview, 15
        P waves, 19–20
        PR interval, 20
        QRS interval, 20–22
        rate, 16–18
        rhythm, 15–16
    mechanical events, 4–5
    overview, 1
    QT interval, 22–23
    T wave, 22
    U wave, 22
    (See also specific types of ECG by
        name)
18-lead ECG, 266
Electrical conduction pathway, of
    heart:
    atrioventricular node, 8
    bundle branches, 8
    bundle of His, 8
    interatrial pathway, 7
    internodal pathway, 7
    overview, 6–7
    Purkinje fibers, 8
    sinoatrial node, 7
Electrocardiogram (see ECG)
Electrolyte changes:
    calcium: hypercalcemia, 243–248
        hypocalcemia, 239–243
        overview, 237–238
    depolarization/repolarization
        process, 1

Electrolyte changes (Cont.):
    magnesium: hypermagnesemia,
        233–237
        hypomagnesemia, 229–233
        overview, 229
    potassium: hyperkalemia, 221–228
        hypokalemia, 215–221
        overview, 215
Electromechanical dissociation (EMD),
    152
Emboli, 74, 76
EMD (electromechanical dissociation),
    152
Endocardium, 5
Enhanced automaticity, 47, 66
Epicardial pacemakers, 286
Epicardium, 5
Epinephrine:
    bradycardia treatment with, 304
    hyperkalemia and, 226
    pulseless arrest, 308
    pulseless electrical activity, 155
    sinus bradycardia and, 32
    ventricular tachycardia, 143
Epinephrine, vasopressin, amiodarone,
    lidocaine (EVAL), 150
Escape rhythms, 23, 119
ESWL (extracorporeal shock wave
    lithotripsy), 292
EVAL (epinephrine, vasopressin,
    amiodarone, lidocaine), 150
Excitability, 2–3
Excretion methods, potassium, 226
External pulse generator box, 298
Extracorporeal shock wave lithotripsy
    (ESWL), 292
Extrasystolic beats, 2, 103–104, 192–193

F
Fail-safe beats, 84, 118
Fetal conduction pathways, 108
Fibrinolytics, 275
15-lead ECG, 266
Fine atrial fibrillation, 75
Fine ventricular fibrillation, 149f
First-degree heart block (1° HB):
    assessment of, 165
    care measures for, 166–167
    causes of, 164–165
    interpretation criteria, 165–166
    overview, 163–164
Five-leadwire system, 10, 11f
Fixed rate pacemakers, 287

Flat line, 156
  (*See also* Asystole)
Flatline artifact, 25*f*
Fluid boluses, 276
Fluid overload, 66
Focal atrial tachycardia, 58
Furosemide:
  hypercalcemia and, 248
  hyperkalemia and, 228*t*

G
Gastrointestinal bleeding, 253
Glycoprotein IIb/IIIa inhibitors, 277
Granulomatous diseases, 244
Grid measurements, 17*f*

H
Healing phase, MI, 252
Heart anatomy, 5*f*
Heart rate (*see* Rate)
Heart–fatty acid-binding protein,
    257
Hemodialysis, 226, 236
Hemodynamic instability:
  atrial fibrillation, 76
  atrial rhythms, 79
  junctional tachycardia, 100
Hemodynamic stability:
  accelerated idioventricular rhythm,
    136
  atrial rhythms, 79
Hemopneumothorax, 255
Hypercalcemia:
  assessment of, 245–246
  care measures for, 247–248
  causes of, 244–245
  interpretation criteria, 246–247
  overview, 243–244
Hyperkalemia:
  assessment of, 223–224
  care measures for, 225–228
  causes of, 221–223
  interpretation criteria, 224–225
  overview, 221
  Wenckebach, 168
Hypermagnesemia:
  assessment of, 234–235
  care measures for, 236–237
  causes of, 234
  interpretation criteria, 235–236
  overview, 233–234
Hyperparathyroidism, 244

Hypocalcemia:
  assessment of, 240–241
  care measures for, 242–243
  causes of, 239–240
  hypomagnesemia and, 231
  interpretation criteria, 242
  overview, 239
Hypokalemia:
  assessment of, 217–218
  care measures for, 219–221
  causes of, 216–217
  interpretation criteria,
    218–219
  overview, 215–216
Hypomagnesemia:
  assessment of, 231
  care measures for, 233
  causes of, 230–231
  interpretation criteria, 232
  overview, 229–230
Hypoparathyroidism, 239
Hypothermia, 119
Hypovolemia, 153
Hypoxia, 153

I
IABP (intra-aortic balloon pump),
    277–278
Ibutilide, 70
ICD (Implantable Cardioverter-
    Defibrillator), 299–300
Idioventricular rhythm (IVR):
  assessment of, 130
  care measures for, 132
  causes of, 129–130
  heart rate and, 23, 213
  interpretation criteria, 130–131
  overview, 128–129
IMA (ischemia-modified albumin), 257
Implantable Cardioverter-Defibrillator
    (ICD), 299–300
Incomplete AV block, 163
Indigestion, 255, 270
Infarction chest pain, 255
Infarction stage, 264–265
Inferior wall myocardial infarction,
    269–270
Injury stage, MI, 262–263
Insulin, 216, 222, 227*t*
Interatrial pathway, 7
Internodal pathway, 7
Interpolated PVC, 125*f*

Interpretation method:
  overview, 15, 189
  P waves, 19–20
  PR interval, 20
  QRS interval, 20–22
  rate, 16–18
  rhythm, 15–16
Intra-aortic balloon pump (IABP),
    277–278
Intravenous calcium, 226
Intravenous potassium, 219–221
Inverted P′ waves, 91–92, 96
Irregular narrow-complex tachycardia, 306
Irregular pulse, 86
Irregular rhythms, 204–207
Irritability beats, 119
Ischemia stage, 260–262
Ischemia-modified albumin (IMA), 257
Isoelectric line, 20
IVR (see Idioventricular rhythm)

J
JER (see Junctional escape rhythm)
JT (see Junctional tachycardia)
Junctional escape focus, 178
Junctional escape rhythm (JER):
  assessment of, 91
  care measures for, 93
  causes of, 90
  dysrhythmias and, 23
  interpretation criteria, 91–92
  overview, 89
Junctional rhythms:
  accelerated: assessment of, 95
    care measures for, 97
    causes of, 94–95
    interpretation criteria, 96
    overview, 94
  AV nodal reentrant tachycardia:
    assessment of, 104–105
    care measures for, 106–107
    causes of, 103–104
    interpretation criteria, 105
    overview, 102–103
  AV reentrant tachycardia: assessment
    of, 109
    care measures for, 111–112
    causes of, 108–109
    interpretation criteria, 109–111
    overview, 107–108
  comparison of, 112–115
  differentiating, 191t

Junctional rhythms (Cont.):
  junctional escape rhythm:
    assessment of, 91
    care measures for, 93
    causes of, 90
    interpretation criteria, 91–92
    overview, 89
  junctional tachycardia: assessment
    of, 99–100
    care measures for, 101–102
    causes of, 98–99
    interpretation criteria, 100–101
    overview, 98
  overview, 83
  premature junctional contractions:
    assessment of, 86
    care measures for, 88–89
    causes of, 84–86
    interpretation criteria, 87–88
    overview, 84
Junctional tachycardia (JT):
  assessment of, 99–100
  care measures for, 101–102
  causes of, 98–99
  interpretation criteria, 100–101
  overview, 98
Junctional tissue, 8

K
Kayexalate, 226, 228t

L
Large box countdown method, 18–19
Lasix, 228t
Lateral wall myocardial infarction,
    271–272
LBBB (left bundle branch block), 181,
    184f
Leads:
  augmented, 9
  contiguous, 260–261
  involvement at myocardial infarction
    sites, 266f, 267t
  limb, 9
  placement, 13–14t
Left bundle branch block (LBBB), 181,
    184f
Lidocaine, 150, 308
Location sites:
  differentiation of rhythms by, 190–191
  myocardial infarction: anterior wall,
    267–269

Location sites, myocardial infarction:
anterior wall (*Cont.*):
inferior wall, 269–270
lateral wall, 271–272
overview, 265–267
posterior wall, 273–274
septal wall, 272–273
Loop diuretics:
hypokalemia and, 216
hypomagnesemia and, 230
premature junctional contractions
and, 84

M
Magnesium:
dietary sources of, 233
hypermagnesemia: assessment of,
234–235
care measures for, 236–237
causes of, 234
interpretation criteria, 235–236
overview, 233–234
hypomagnesemia: assessment of,
231
care measures for, 233
causes of, 230–231
interpretation criteria, 232
overview, 229–230
overview, 229
pulseless arrest, 308
replacement, 54
Magnesium sulfate, 233
Magnetic resonance imaging (MRI), 292
Magnets, pacemakers, 297
MAT (multi-focal atrial tachycardia),
58–59, 62
Mechanical events, 4–5
MI (*see* Myocardial infarction)
Microshocks, pacemaker, 298
Mithramycin, 248
Mobitz, Woldemar, 167
Modifiable risk factors, MI, 253
MONA mnemonic, 275
Monomorphic premature ventricular
contractions, 122*f*
Monomorphic ventricular tachycardia,
140*f*
Morphine, 276
Mouth-to-mouth resuscitation, 151
MRI (magnetic resonance imaging), 292
Multi-focal atrial tachycardia (MAT),
58–59, 62

Multifocal premature ventricular
contractions, 122*f*
Multi-formed atrial rhythm, 55
Muscle strain, 255
Muscular artifact, 25*f*
Myocardial contusion, 255
Myocardial infarction (MI), 251–280
care measures for, 275–279
causes of, 252–254
chest pain, 256*t*
diagnosis of: history, 254–256
physical assessment, 254–256
serum cardiac markers,
257–258
interpretation criteria: location sites,
265–274
stages of damage, 259–265
overview, 251
Myocardium, 5
Myoglobin, 258*t*

N
Narrow complex tachycardia, 153
Narrow QRS waves, 207–212
NASPE/BPG (North American Society
of Pacing and
Electrophysiology/British
Pacing and Electrophysiology
Group), 287–288
Neuromuscular excitability, 231
Neuromuscular transmission blockage,
234
Nitroglycerin, 276
Nonconducted premature atrial
contraction, 52*f*
Nonmodifiable risk factors, MI, 253
Non-Q wave myocardial infarction,
264
Nonrespiratory sinus dysrhythmia,
38–39
Nonsustained ventricular tachycardia,
140
Norepinephrine, 6
Normal depolarization (*see* Antegrade
depolarization)
Normal sinus rhythm (NSR), 27–28
North American Society of Pacing and
Electrophysiology and British
Pacing and Electrophysiology
Group (NASPE/BPEG),
287–288
NSR (normal sinus rhythm), 27–28

O

Occlusion of coronary arteries, 251
Oral potassium supplements, 219
Organic heart disease, 55
Orthodromic reentrant tachycardia, 107
Oxygen therapy, 275

P

P waves:
 atrial rhythms and, 47
 bundle branches and, 172
 overview, 19–20
 sinus rhythm, 27
 sinus tachycardia, 197
P' waves:
 atrial flutter, 197
 atrial rhythms and, 47–48
 atrial tachycardia, 58–59, 61, 197
 AVNRT and AVRT, 198
 inverted, 91–92, 96
 wandering atrial pacemaker, 56
PAC (*see* Premature atrial contractions)
Pacemaker spike, 290
Pacemakers:
 care measures after: permanent insertion, 296–297
  temporary placement, 298–299
 Implantable Cardioverter-Defibrillator, 299–300
 interference with function of, 291–293
 interpretation criteria, 290–291
 length of use, 283
 malfunction of: failure to capture, 294
  failure to pace, 293–294
  failure to sense, 295
  oversensing, 295–296
 myocardial infarctions and, 278
 rationale for, 281–282
 routes for: epicardial, 286
  transcutaneous, 283–285
  transvenous, 286
 settings for, 286–290
 sources interfering with, 293t
 types of, 282
Palpitations, 86, 120
Pancreatitis:
 acute, 230
 hypocalcemia and, 239
Paper technique, 16

Parasympathetic nervous system, 6
Parasympathetic stimulation, 3
Parathyroid gland, 239
Parathyroid hormones, 238
Paroxysmal atrial fibrillation, 72
Paroxysmal supraventricular tachycardia, 102
Pathologic Q waves, 264
PEA (*see* Pulseless electrical activity)
Percutaneous coronary interventions, 278
Percutaneous transluminal coronary angioplasty (PTCA), 277
Pericardial sac, 5
Pericarditis, 255
Peritoneal dialysis, 236–237
Permanent pacemaker insertion, 283, 296–297
Persistent atrial fibrillation, 72
Phosphate binders, 243
PJC (*see* Premature junctional contractions)
Plateau phase (Phase 2), 1
Pneumothorax, 255
Polymorphic premature ventricular contractions, 122f
Polymorphic ventricular tachycardia, 140, 141f
Posterior wall myocardial infarction, 273–274
Potassium:
 hyperkalemia: assessment of, 223–224
  care measures for, 225–228
  causes of, 221–223
  interpretation criteria, 224–225
  overview, 221
 hypokalemia: assessment of, 217–218
  care measures for, 219–221
  causes of, 216–217
  interpretation criteria, 218–219
  overview, 215–216
 overview, 215
 replacement, 54
PQRST complexes, 212
P'R interval, 50, 56, 87
PR interval (PRI), 20, 173–174
Precordial leads, 9
Pre-excitation syndromes, 108
Pre-excited atrial fibrillation, 306
Preload, 5

Premature atrial contractions (PAC):
  assessment of, 49–50
  care measures for, 53–54
  causes of, 48–49
  interpretation criteria, 50–53
  overview, 48
Premature junctional contractions (PJC):
  assessment of, 86
  care measures for, 88–89
  causes of, 84–86
  interpretation criteria, 87–88
  overview, 84
Premature ventricular contractions
      (PVCs):
  assessment of, 120–121
  care measures for, 127–128
  causes of, 119–120
  interpretation criteria, 121–127
  overview, 117–118
PRI (PR interval), 20, 173–174
Procainamide:
  PJCs and, 85
  Wolff–Parkinson–White syndrome,
      111
PTCA (percutaneous transluminal
      coronary angioplasty), 277
Pulse deficit, 74
Pulse generator, 285
Pulseless arrest algorithm, 143, 308
Pulseless electrical activity (PEA):
  assessment of, 153–154
  care measures for, 155–156
  causes of, 153
  interpretation criteria, 154–155
  overview, 152
Pulseless rhythms, 213–214
Pulseless ventricular tachycardia, 147
Purkinje fibers, 8
PVCs (see Premature ventricular
      contractions)

Q
Q wave, 20–21
Q wave MI, 264
QRS interval (QRS I), 20–22
QRS waves:
  narrow versus wide, 207–213
  ratio of P waves to, 20
  tachycardia algorithm, 306
QT interval, 22–23
Quadrigeminal premature ventricular
      contractions, 123f

"Quick and dirty" countdown method, 19
Quinidine, 84–85

R
R waves, 21, 109, 180, 183
"Rabbit-ear" formation, 180, 183
Radiofrequency catheter ablation, 77,
      106, 111, 292
Rapid repolarization, 1–2
Rapid ventricular response (RVR), 68, 75f
Rate:
  accelerated idioventricular rhythm
      and, 213
  idioventricular rhythm and, 213
  large box countdown method,
      18–19
  overview, 16–18
  pacemakers and, 286
  "quick and dirty" countdown
      method, 19
  small box countdown method, 18
  temperature, body and, 34
  ventricular tachycardia and, 213
Rate control therapy, 79
Rate-responsive pacemakers, 282
RBBB (right bundle branch block),
      180, 184f
Reentrant atrial tachycardia, 58–59
Reentry mechanisms, 24
Reentry supraventricular tachycardia, 306
Refractoriness, 3–4
Regular rhythms, 198–204
Relative refractory period, 4
Reperfusion treatment, 185
Repolarization, 1–2
Resonance sinus dysrhythmia, 38–39
Resting phase, 2
Resynchronization therapy, 281
Retrograde depolarization, 84, 89, 94, 98
Rhythm control therapy, 79
Rhythms:
  differentiation of: bradycardia versus
      tachycardia, 193–198
    extrasystolic beats, 192–193
    by location site, 190–191
    narrow versus wide QRS waves,
      207–213
    pulseless rhythms, 213–214
    regular versus irregular, 198–207
  overview, 15–16
  pulseless arrest algorithm, 308
  tachycardia algorithm, 306

Right bundle branch block (RBBB), 180, 184*f*
R-on-T phenomenon, 124, 125*f*
R-R interval, 84
Runs, 122–123, 124*f*
RVR (rapid ventricular response), 68, 75*f*

S
SA (*see* Sinoatrial arrest)
SA node, 2, 7, 41
Salvos, 122–123, 124*f*
Sarcoidosis, 244
SB (*see* Sinus bradycardia)
SD (*see* Sinus dysrhythmia)
Second-degree heart block (2° HB):
    Mobitz 2°: assessment of, 173
        care measures for, 175–176
        causes of, 172–173
        interpretation criteria, 173–175
        overview, 172
    Wenckebach: assessment of, 169
        care measures for, 171
        causes of, 168–169
        interpretation criteria, 169–171
        overview, 167–168
Septal wall myocardial infarction, 272–273
Serum cardiac markers, 257–258
Shortened diastole, 60
Single-chamber pacemakers, 282
Sinoatrial (SA) node, 2, 7, 41
Sinoatrial arrest (SA):
    assessments of, 42–44
    care measures for, 44–45
    junctional rhythms and, 83
    overview, 41
Sinus block, 83
Sinus bradycardia (SB):
    assessments of, 30–31
    care measures for, 31–32
    causes of, 29–30
    junctional rhythms and, 83
    overview, 28–29
Sinus dysrhythmia (SD):
    assessments of, 39–40
    care measures for, 40–41
    causes of, 38–39
    overview, 38
Sinus rhythms:
    comparison of, 45
    differentiating, 191*t*

Sinus rhythms (*Cont.*):
    normal, 21*f*, 27–28
    sinoatrial arrest: assessments of, 42–44
        care measures for, 44–45
        causes of, 42
        overview, 41
    sinus bradycardia: assessments of, 30–31
        care measures for, 31–32
        causes of, 29–30
        overview, 28–29
    sinus dysrhythmia: assessments of, 39–40
        care measures for, 40–41
        causes of, 38–39
        overview, 38
    sinus tachycardia: assessments of, 35–37
        care measures for, 37–38
        causes of, 33–35
        overview, 32–33
Sinus tachycardia (ST):
    assessments of, 35–37
    care measures for, 37–38
    causes of, 33–35
    overview, 32–33
    P waves, 197
    segment depression, 260–261, 273–274
    segment elevation, 262–263
6-second strip, 19
60-cycle electrical interference, 25*f*
Small box countdown method, 18
SNS (sympathetic nervous system) stimulation, 6, 33
Sodium bicarbonate, 226
Sodium polystyrene sulfonate, 228*t*
ST (*see* Sinus tachycardia)
Stroke volume, 5
Subendocardial infarction, 259
Supernormal refractory period, 4
Supraventricular tachycardia (SVT), 36, 63, 196–197, 306
Sympathetic nervous system (SNS) stimulation, 6, 33
Sympathetic stimulation, 3
Symptomatic Mobitz block, 176
Symptomatic rhythm, PVC, 127
Symptomatic sinus bradydysrhythmia, 40
Synchronized cardioversion, 77, 106
Synchronous pacing, 295

T

T waves, 4, 22
  hyperkalemia and, 224
  inversion, 261
Tachycardia, 196–198, 306
Tachycardia with pulses algorithm,
    70, 77, 306
Tachycardic rhythms, 200–201t
TEE (transesophageal
    echocardiogram), 70, 77
Temperature, body, 34
Temporary pacemaker placement,
    283, 298–299
TENS (transcutaneous electrical nerve
    stimulator), 292
Tension pneumothorax, 255
Thiazide diuretics:
  hypercalcemia and, 244, 248
  hypokalemia and, 216
  hypomagnesemia and, 230
  PJCs and, 84
Third-degree heart block (3° HB):
  assessment of, 177–178
  care measures for, 180
  causes of, 177
  interpretation criteria, 178–179
  overview, 176–177
Three-lead system, 10f
Thrombolytic therapy, 277
Toad venom ingestion, 222
Torsades de pointes, 138, 306
Transcutaneous electrical nerve
    stimulator (TENS), 292
Transcutaneous pacemakers,
    180, 283–285
Transcutaneous pacing, 32, 136, 175, 304
Transesophageal echocardiogram (TEE),
    70, 77
Transvenous pacemakers, 185, 286, 304
Trigeminal premature ventricular
    contractions, 123f
Triggered activity, 24, 47
Troponin I, 258t
Troponin T, 258t
Trousseau's sign, 241f
Tuberculosis, 244
12-lead ECG:
  atrial flutter and, 70
  defined, 1
  diagnosing myocardial infarction
    sites, 266
  electrode placement, 12f
  overview, 8–9
  procedure, 9–14

2° HB (see Second-degree heart block)
2:1 Mobitz block, 174
Type I atrial flutter, 66, 68
Type II atrial flutter, 66, 68

U

U wave, 22
Unifocal premature ventricular
    contractions, 122f

V

VAD (ventricular assist device), 278
Vagal maneuvers:
  atrial flutter and, 70
  AV nodal reentrant tachycardia, 106
Vasopressin, 143–144, 308
Ventolin, 227t
Ventricular assist device (VAD), 278
Ventricular escape focus, 178
Ventricular fibrillation (VF):
  assessment of, 147–148
  care measures for, 149–151
  causes of, 147
  interpretation criteria, 148–149
  overview, 146
Ventricular paced, sensed, and inhibited
    pacemaker (VVI),
    288–289
Ventricular regularity, 16
Ventricular rhythms, 117–162
  accelerated idioventricular rhythm:
    assessment of, 134
    care measures for, 136–137
    causes of, 133–134
    interpretation criteria, 135–136
    overview, 133
  asystole: assessment of, 158–159
    care measures for, 160
    causes of, 157–158
    interpretation criteria, 159
    overview, 156–157
  comparison of, 160–161
  differentiating, 191t
  idioventricular rhythm: assessment
    of, 130
    care measures for, 132
    causes of, 129–130
    interpretation criteria,
      130–131
    overview, 128–129
  premature ventricular contractions:
    assessment of, 120–121
    care measures for, 127–128
    causes of, 119–120

Ventricular rhythms, premature
    ventricular contractions:
        assessment of *(Cont.)*:
    interpretation criteria, 121–127
    overview, 117–118
    pulseless electrical activity:
        assessment of, 153–154
        care measures for, 155–156
        causes of, 153
        interpretation criteria, 154–155
        overview, 152
    ventricular fibrillation: assessment
        of, 147–148
        care measures for, 149–151
        causes of, 147
        interpretation criteria, 148–149
        overview, 146
    ventricular tachycardia: assessment
        of, 139
        care measures for, 142–145
        causes of, 138–139
        interpretation criteria, 140–142
        overview, 137
Ventricular standstill, 159
Ventricular tachycardia (VT):
    assessment of, 139
    care measures for, 142–145

Ventricular tachycardia (VT) *(Cont.)*:
    causes of, 138–139
    heart rate and, 213
    interpretation criteria, 140–142
    overview, 137
    tachycardia algorithm, 306
Vessels, MI, 266f, 267t
VF (*see* Ventricular fibrillation)
VOO mode, pacing, 295
VT (*see* Ventricular tachycardia)
VVI (ventricular paced, sensed, and
        inhibited pacemaker), 288–289

W
Wandering atrial pacemaker (WAP):
    assessment of, 56
    care measures for, 57–58
    causes of, 55–56
    interpretation criteria, 56–57
    overview, 55
Wandering baseline, 25f
Wenckebach, Karel, 167
Wenckebach block, 52, 195t
Wide QRS waves, 212–213
"Widow-maker," 268
Wolff–Parkinson–White (WPW)
        syndrome, 107